"Out of the approximate 2.5 million deaths in the U.S. annually, only 14,000 are suitable organ donors. For this reason, we need to cast the net wide so that we capture those precious few to save many."

—Cathy Olmo
CTDN's Community Affairs Volunteer Coordinator
(California and Nevada)

"Living and deceased organ donation is a generous and emotional sacrifice and gift that has a transforming impact on the lives of others. The inspirational stories of these donors and their families need to be told. They are true heroes."

—Marc L. Melcher, M.D., Ph.D.
Assistant Professor, Multi-organ Transplantation,
Department of Surgery, Stanford University Medical Center,
Lucille Packard Children's Hospital

"A GIFT NOT WASTED is engaging and filled with such strong emotions and family bonds. Giving the gift of life created a passion for continuing to share your story, which educates people about organ donation."

—Amy S. Peele, RN
Director of Transplant Clinical Operations,
University of California, San Francisco Medical Center

A Gift Not Wasted

A Memoir

Belia Marina

Durban House

Copyright © 2009, Belia M. Rennels

All rights reserved. No part of this book may be used or
reproduced in any manner whatsoever without
the written permission of the Publisher.

Printed in the United States of America.

For information address:

Durban House Press, Inc.
5001 LBJ Freeway, Suite 700
Dallas, Texas 75244

Library of Congress Cataloging-in-Publication Data

Rennels, Belia M.

A Gift Not Wasted/Belia M. Rennels

Library of Congress Control Number: 2008934979

p. cm.

ISBN: 978-0-9818486-1-7

First Edition

10 9 8 7 6 5 4 3 2 1

Visit our Web site at
http://www.durbanhouse.com

In loving memory of

Sylvia Marina Zertuche

Acknowledgments

I acknowledge the dedication and skill of the University of San Francisco Medical Center's Kidney Transplant Services and its entire staff, particularly noted nephrologist Dr. William Amend (ret.), who granted me an interview; Dr. Juliet Melzer, my surgeon; Transplant Coordinator Ana Marie Torres; and the incredible ICU nursing staff. To Kaiser Permanente, for making sure Sylvia received the best medical care available. Special thanks to my wonderful daughter Cynthia, who awakened me to the fact that I could be a kidney donor. Deep love and appreciation to my husband, Don, and son, Joe, on whom I relied for emotional support during the time described in this book and still do today.

A note of thanks to my extended family, the Zertuches, and to the Zaragoza family, who generously shared the inspiring story of their son Matthew with me. To the National Kidney Foundation and the California Transplant Donor Network for their continual efforts in educating the public on our ability to save lives. Most of all, thanks to my editor, Bob Middlemiss, the man who guided me through the process of telling my story effectively. His faith in this work and his insistence for me to dig deeper are reflected on every page.

You give but little when you give of your possessions. It is when you give of yourself that you truly give.

—Kahlil Gibran

Introduction

This story takes place within my Mexican-American family, who, like many other ethnic groups, have blended the best of two cultures. While ferociously proud of being Americans, we retain our Mexican heritage, cherishing love of family, loyalty and steadfastness above all else. In thick and thin, in joyous and sad times, during exciting and dull moments, we—as the kids say—hang.

You'll read of our customs, music, tools, recreational outlets and the various idiosyncrasies that are present in all family units regardless of origin. Like other families, we endure trials, joys, sadness and whatever life hurls our way. This story zeroes in on a very specific period when our families were young and of the extraordinary circumstance that called upon the strength of our love. It chronicles our family's response to what we perceived as a catastrophe, but one which we knew we would weather together because that's what our family did. With God's help, we tapped into our deepest reserves to rally around one of our children when she was faced with a life-threatening challenge.

To fully appreciate the intertwining of our lives, it's necessary to describe Sylvia's and my relationship as godchild and godmother. That relationship in our Mexican culture is bound by extremely strong traditions that give it a very special status. For instance, godchildren address godparents as *nino* (short for *padrino*) and *nina* (short for *madrina*). The child's parents and the couple they choose to baptize their infant become *compadre* (co-father) and *comadre* (co-mother). As the titles imply, godparents are held in high esteem because they bear the responsibility of their godchild's welfare, both physical and spiritual, should anything happen to the parents.

From the date of the baptism, the parents and godparents no longer refer to one another by first names, but only by the titles that respect their alliance. To me, Sylvia's father was *compadre*, or *compadre* Armando. Her mother was *comadre* or *comadre* Maggie. I, to them, was *comadre*. To their daughter, Sylvia, I was simply *nina*.

For those who honor the commitment (and there are varying degrees of observance), being a godparent within our Mexican tradition is a privilege as well as an obligation. This relationship is the foundation of the story. It explains the reason Sylvia's crisis impacted us, her godparents, as well as the rest of the family as deeply as it did. My children considered her a sister, as did most of her cousins. My brothers-in-law and their wives looked upon her as a second daughter.

When my niece and godchild, Sylvia, suffered chronic kidney failure at eighteen, our family drew upon this fundamental tradition to cope with the crisis. It was a strange journey through an unfamiliar world of nephrologists (kidney specialists), dialysis, organ donation, organ waiting lists and kidney transplantation. We rallied around Sylvia and her parents. Despite our deep faith in God, our underlying fear was that the solution seemed beyond our ability to achieve.

When we fully digest the impact of what kidney failure means, we're chilled with the prospect that love may be insufficient to conquer the challenge. However, love did prevail in the form of Terri, Sylvia's older sister. Terri donated her kidney to Sylvia for her first transplant. Suddenly, our lives were back on course as we celebrated the success of the transplant surgery. Our jubilation lulled us into believing that our Sylvia was home free. As we basked in the triumph, we never considered that victories are often short-lived.

Eleven years later, the transplanted kidney reached the end of its life expectancy, and Sylvia's body went into rejection. Sylvia's plight repeated itself. Again we found the solution amongst ourselves. I gave Sylvia her second kidney. The surgery was successful, the joint recuperation period rewarding and often humorous. Those four weeks of joint convalescence remain a cherished memory indelibly tattooed in every fiber of my being. This second victory infused us with confidence that the threat had truly been conquered that time. For six months, our family breathed a collective sigh of relief. To our horror, at the end of that time, catastrophe struck again, and despite an overwhelming outpouring of love, it was not enough to save Sylvia a third time.

Everyone, especially my *comadre* and her family, dealt with Sylvia's loss as best they could. For me it meant struggling to understand how such a tragic end could have happened. Within a week of her death, I listed a chronology of Sylvia's last few weeks. I reasoned that perhaps by better understanding these events, my sorrow would lessen. When I finished it, I put it away. But it never left me. I thought of it every day, picturing where it was tucked away, knowing each word by heart and promising myself that someday soon I'd retrieve it and turn it into a story. As I drove home from work, shopped or watched TV in the evening, it hibernated in the back of my mind. Sometimes, I'd start for the cabinet where it was buried, but couldn't bring myself to hold it, read it or bear the remembrance.

I'll never know what changes occurred within me to reverse that pattern, but about two years later I did pull it out. Coffee mug in hand, I skimmed the facts that I knew by memory. Halfway through the chronology, my eyes clouded with tears and I tossed it back into the cabinet. This time it only took a few months before I found the resolve to dig it out again. Then I began this book in earnest. I still wonder whether I'll ever get through some of the parts without my throat thickening or eyes welling up.

Once I started the book, I also decided to volunteer for the National Kidney Foundation, hoping that involving myself in their good work might be another means to deal with the loss. Shortly after volunteering for the NKF, I learned of the California Transplant Donor Network and began volunteering for that group. It wasn't long before I realized that the best way to commemorate Sylvia's life was to encourage organ donation. The more I became involved with both organizations, the more that conviction deepened. The more my commitment grew, the easier it became to transform my grief into a positive, healing process.

Now, in Sylvia's memory, I've become an advocate for organ donation. From that involvement I've learned of many inspiring stories of people who have received organs or people who have been donor families. Undoubtedly, there are many more hundreds of poignant examples that exist. One of the most exemplary cases of what donating life to others can mean stems from an interview I was granted by the Zaragoza family of Manteca, California. The last chapter is devoted to their sixteen-year-old, Matthew, who died in 2005, and to them as an incredibly selfless family. It is a privilege to describe and acknowledge the tremendous love that saved the lives of four people. Their story will amaze you.

The topic of organ donation may not appeal to some, but I can guarantee you that if one of your family members or a loved one was placed on an organ waiting list that presently averages six years, you would reconsider this option. And that is what it is—an option. Only you can judge whether it is right for you. Perhaps when you learn what donating life truly means, you may subscribe to that life-saving ability we're all capable of granting. I sincerely hope so.

The following pages will depict how one Mexican-American family gathered together in a time of crisis by responding with all the love they could muster to grapple with a horrendous reality. It was a time when we felt our oneness as never before or since. It is Sylvia's legacy that she bound us tighter as a family during a difficult time. She is the inspiration of this memoir.

1

Corridor of Memories

San Francisco's Sunset Boulevard was as black and cold as our spirits. I'd never driven it at four-thirty in the morning, but the tree-lined street with its old California Spanish names was still familiar. Why wouldn't it be when, for the past six months, I'd traveled it twice a day, including most weekends? The Buick Skylark practically steered itself as it sped past the familiar sequence of streets: Pacheco, Ortega, Noriega and Moraga toward Judah Street and the climb to Parnassus Hill. It was even too early for the usual morning fog, though traces of its impending arrival haloed the tops of light posts. I knew that by the time the commute hour arrived, the indigenous mist would obscure the white-ribboned lanes along the boulevard.

I knew it without thinking because there was no ability or desire to think. The car moved automatically as I struggled with a mind frozen with anguish. I wouldn't think. I had to resist logic by not thinking, by barricading all thought, because the phone call had to be a lie. It could not be true! If I refused its truth, it would remain untrue.

My niece, Terri, and daughter, Cynthia, rode silently in the rear of the car. We were picking up my *comadre* (who's also my sister-in-law and Terri's mom), Maggie, on the way to the University of San Francisco Medical Center's ICU. She was staying with our niece, Michelle. Ironically, I'd dropped them both off at Michelle's apartment not more than three hours ago.

1

We edged along the curb in front of Michelle's and were barely stopped when Terri leapt from the back seat and headed for the nearest building. Almost immediately, she halted and doubled back. Two silhouettes exited from the entrance of the multiplex that was sandwiched, San Francisco-style, between two other apartment houses. Obviously, they'd been waiting for us. They entered the car without the usual hellos, and the Skylark resumed its route, hauling us along in the silence that marked our common bond of desolation.

It was a few short blocks to Parnassus and the brightly-lit emergency entrance to the hospital. From the entrance booth, a female sentry poked her head out of the framed window, intent on barring any unauthorized entry into the parking lot. I rolled down the car window. Her expression shouted that she was ready to reject whatever reason we'd offer for trespassing into the privileged area of coveted slots.

"We just had a phone call that a family member died." My voice reminded me of Jack Webb's character on the old *Dragnet* television series from the fifties—low, dry, unemotional, factual. Had it really come from me? It felt like a ventriloquist had moved my lips.

Her defensive demeanor melted. With genuine compassion she directed us to park anywhere. After exiting the car, we wordlessly approached the hospital's swooshing double doors that we'd gone through so often of late. This time, they heralded sorrow, not hope. A warren of long passages wound toward a bank of elevators that took us up to another floor with a different bank of elevators. Our footfalls marching on the tiled floors echoed in our ears as we progressed. Patients were still asleep, and personnel moved quietly at five o'clock in the morning.

We melded into this world of hushed inactivity, pushing silently forward. We rounded the last corner that would connect us to the main hospital. The long corridor before us filled me with dread. But there it was, beckoning like a time tunnel. My mind was fogged and bewildered. My heart pounded, and I could almost smell the animal instinct to fight and survive. All faculties were on high alert to deny acceptance of what must not be. We were all mute, tense, terrified, in denial.

Why was this happening? Why, when the second transplant surgery had been so successful? How had we ever gotten trapped in this hideous predicament? I felt the walls close in. As I fought the inner panic, my mind flew backward, back to the beginning, when tiny faces and large expectations filled our hearts. Who would have guessed that a pledge made to a tiny infant could reach such depths? Or scour one's emotional resources? No hint of this had tinged that summer day in 1964.

Sylvia remained sound asleep as the priest anointed her with oils and poured water over her forehead. My then-husband, Jose Guadalupe Zertuche, known as Lupe, and I jointly held her in our arms, tipping her head over the baptismal font at All Souls Church in South San Francisco. The white frilly cap had been removed. The matching lacy gown was unbuttoned at her chubby neck to permit the application of sacred oils. Holy water trickled back over her tilted brow as the priest recited the sacramental words that branded her a child of God. Her wet hair shone bright. Still, she remained asleep.

As Sylvia's godparents, we denounced Satan on her behalf and vowed to watch over her spiritual life. We affirmed that if anything happened to her parents, we would be responsible to ensure that all her needs, spiritual and physical, were met. From this day forward we would be known as her *padrino* and *madrina*, godfather and godmother, though she would eventually shorten the titles to *nino* and *nina*. Maggie and Armando Zertuche, Sylvia's parents, and Lupe and I would henceforth address each other as *compadre* and *comadre*, co-father and co-mother. We'd never use our Christian names when speaking to one another: it would be highly disrespectful to do so.

The relationship between parents, godparents and godchild is very special in the Mexican culture. It's not only an honor to baptize a child; it's a solemn responsibility. As a result, parents give great thought to whom they select for this lifetime obligation and privilege. No one rejects the request to baptize a child, as there is nothing more sacred than new life, nothing more beautiful, holy, or cherished. Refusal is simply out of the question within our Latino world. At least, that's how it was in the sixties.

Maggie and Armando, who was one of Lupe's younger brothers, had asked us to be their second child's godparents several months before Sylvia was born. In 1964, amniocentesis was not the popular procedure it has become today. We didn't know if our godchild would be a boy or a girl. As it turned out, we were delighted to learn that we'd inherited a goddaughter, and I was especially pleased when she was given my middle name.

One year and one day after Sylvia Marina's birthday, our own son was born on June twenty-second. He was named after his father, but we called him Joe. In their early years, Sylvia and our Joe had their birthday parties on the same day, until they entered kindergarten and started cultivating their own little friends. We alternated houses for the parties, and lots of cousins and family friends joined in the fun.

Piñatas were a given. The dads would set up the rope in the backyard from which the colorfully decorated piñata dangled. Blindfolded children swung their sticks in an effort to split it open. The adults squealed as loudly as the children. The piñata bobbed up and down in controlled swoops, ensuring that every child got his turn. With every pitch we oohed and aahed encouragement or disappointment when a swing missed its mark.

Once the break occurred and all the goodies cascaded out, the yard was alive with scrambling kids. Tiny hands scooped up the booty as fast as they could jump from spot to spot. Tangled bodies climbed over one another. Wrapped candies, plastic toys and a few coins were snatched up. Parents yelled, prompting their children, "Over here, over there," as they pointed to plunder still unclaimed. All wanted their children to get their fair share. Inevitably, a little one would end up crying, upset that an older child was more adept at filling his hands and pockets than he was. Comforting adults were always in the wings, waiting to hug. Stray goodies were always found to dry the tears.

Sylvia was one of the quicker kids. Perhaps having had the example of her sister, Terri, who was one year older, gave her an edge. Whatever the reason, Sylvia usually made out quite well in any competitive effort. When she won, her smile was broad and her walk springier than sponge cake. She would tease, "Ha-ha, I got more than you did, Teti" (her nickname for her sister). In the next breath, she'd add, "Want some of mine?"

Before taking Sylvia up on the offer, Teti would get in at least one barb, always delivered with a half-smile. "Hmmph! I think I should, since you knocked me down a couple of times." That might or might not have been true. But delivering a snappy retort among siblings and cousins was picked up from the adults at an early age. It seemed to make life more fun and honed the skills required later for survival in this irascibly funny, tight-knit family.

As we continued traveling through the endless corridor, those events seemed so long ago. The hospital walls crushed in as I obsessed anew on how we had come to such a desolate point. Where had the smiles gone? "Let this cup pass, dear Lord, let it pass," I repeated to myself. Even in my subconscious intercession, I knew what must follow: *Thy will be done.* Yet I couldn't bring myself to accept the second part as we moved down the long corridor toward what awaited us.

2

A Note on Faith

There's no doubt that God was and is an intricate part of our family's life. Faith in our Mexican culture is tremendously important, yet not always conventional. To understand this enigma, as well as our story, I'll try to explain how our faith is reflected in our lives.

We all know that the world sometimes customizes religion, faith, and belief in God to comfortably fit a lifestyle. In addition, there's a tendency to consider these attributes as wonderful as long as they aren't inconvenient. Some are more faithful to the letter of their faith (church/temple/mosque/other) and obey whatever precepts of worship their faith requires. In the eighties and nineties, the Zertuches held God and faith in a special, revered niche that rarely interfered with their way of life. This was also typical with other Mexican families, as well as non-Mexican ones.

Yes, the crucifix hung in their homes, and a picture of Our Lady of Guadalupe was an absolute given. Votive candles placed before religious statues or holy pictures were as normal as the kitchen fixtures. A rosary might hang on a corner of the frame of a holy picture as decoration, but it was rarely, if ever, used in prayer. I doubt whether anyone knew the names of each of the five decades, which are the groupings of ten beads separated by a space followed by a single bead representing the place when the Our Father, or Lord's Prayer, is recited. By the way, we say it's the Our Father, while others refer to it as the Lord's Prayer—either way, it's the same prayer. The beginning of each rosary decade is called a "mystery" and named for a significant event in the life of either Jesus or Mary. That information might or might not have been known in my in-laws' houses, nor was it considered relevant.

Most Mexican families are Catholic; we are Catholic. But, with the exception of my *comadre*, Maggie, my husband, children and me, no one else attended Mass on a regular basis. Neither were the others members of the so-called "Christmas-Easter Catholics" club that is so frustratingly referred to from the pulpit by the clergy. They attended church when their children received the sacraments of Baptism, Holy Communion and Confirmation, as well as for weddings or funerals of family and friends. For the most part, the men preferred to skip the nuptial Mass in favor of simply attending the wedding reception.

Did this casual treatment of their religion mean that they didn't have faith? Didn't believe in God? The very thought of such an idea would have generated angry denials by everyone normally seated around my mother-in-law's kitchen table. They loved God and had a deep, abiding faith in the Almighty. Their faith coursed through their veins with every heartbeat and in every breath.

Typically, everyday speech in Latino families reflects our relationship with God. Everyone knows that *"adios"* means "go with God." Whenever we make plans for the following day, it's common to say, *"Si Dios nos da vida, mañana hasemos…"* (If God grants us life, tomorrow we'll do…). When a person sneezes, one says *"Jesus le ayude"* (Jesus help you). Something I always find funny is that on the rare occasion when no one offers the *"Jesus le ayude"* bit, the sneezer snaps back with, *"Jesus me ayude mientras llego donde hay gente."* Translation: "Jesus help me until I get to where there are (civilized) people." This indicates how rude the lack of the proper response is considered to be.

When asked if we're planning on going somewhere or doing something in particular, we answer with *"Dios dira,"* which means "God will decide." Whenever the name of a deceased person is mentioned, the words *"En pas descanse"* ("may he/she rest in peace") quickly follow. The reference implies the wish that the person be in heaven with God, our

Father. When we state that we hope to see someone again, we respond with *"Dios primero."* The literal translation is "God first," but really means "if it's His will."

These and many other phrases that acknowledge God's presence and authority are so engrained in our everyday conversation that it's considered discourteous not to use them at the appropriate times. Additionally, their generous use is a barometer of good manners. It is an assumed fact that He is intricately present in our lives. When troubled with problems, ill health or the type of tragedy that engulfed us during Sylvia's illness, you can bet God's mercy was invoked by every member of the household.

A common sight that I witnessed when visiting the Basilica of Our Lady of Guadalupe in Mexico City many years ago was that of a long line of faithful inching along on their knees on cobbled stones. The self-inflicted torment is an offering or sacrifice to merit an answer to a prayer or as thanksgiving for having had one answered. It can also be an act of contrition and plea for forgiveness.

This calls to mind another custom typical of our culture. It deals with making a *"demanda,"* or demand from God. There's quite a variation on this practice, but basically it's making a request of God or of Our Lady with the promise that if it's granted, we will comply with whatever they demand. Curiously, we also make up the demand (or method of payback) ourselves. It must be a substantial offering of personal sacrifice.

For instance, if someone needs a job, he (or she) might pray for it and promise that if he gets the job, he will say a certain number of rosaries, do a novena (nine days of prayer), attend so many Masses, or donate a particular sum to the church. If someone has undergone testing for a serious ailment, he might pray for negative results, or if he is truly ill, that he be cured. If his pleas are answered, he might make a pledge, or *demanda*, to make a special pilgrimage to a certain shrine. Invoking the use of a *demanda* is usually reserved for heavy-duty needs. But this practice is one more example that demonstrates the zealous faith that's part of our lives. These examples were second nature to the Zertuches, who, without question, believe. I know of at least one of my brothers-in-law who placed a *demanda* before God, and I suspect some of the others did also.

Oftentimes the only jewelry you see a Mexican man wear is a chain with a crucifix or with a medallion of Our Lady of Guadalupe. Many women wear the cross or medals along with their regular jewelry. Cars will have these same objects dangling from the rearview mirror, or a rosary or a combination of all three. Are they lucky charms or reminders of the faith? Probably a combination of both.

Obviously, there are atheists and agnostics in every country, and there must be Mexicans who fall into those categories. Yet I've never met a Mexican or known of one who doesn't subscribe to the practices mentioned above.

Although the majority of our family didn't attend Mass, they felt, acknowledged and trusted in God's presence. Like wayward children who know that their parents love them unconditionally, they knew that God loved them and that they were His children. It was an indisputable reality.

Normally, the Mexican mother is the upholder of the faith within her family. The father expects it and supports it. She ensures that their children are taught the catechism of the Catholic faith and receive the sacraments. Not so in the Zertuche household. Maria might have been spiritual in her way, but she was not visibly religious. Still, she did believe in God, invoked his name, occasionally prayed, and required that her children and grandchildren be baptized. On occasion she might light a candle in her home for a special intention. However, she rarely went to church other than to attend weddings, *quinceañeras* (a girl's 15th birthday coming-out party) or funerals. Even those attendances were kept to a minimum. It was not her practice to flaunt her faith. She preferred to keep it buried in her bosom, yet we all knew it existed.

Matias, my father-in-law, was of the same mind as his wife but even more respectful, and especially guarded against using God's name in vain or doubting His authority. He used to tell the story of one of his brothers who was smitten by God for his arrogance. During his youth in his home town of Cloete, his older brother, Gregorio, had become very rich through ownership in a chain of movie houses. Vainly proud of his good fortune, Gregorio was heard to boast (in Spanish), "I'm so wealthy that not even God can make me poor!" He ended up dying penniless in his middle-aged years.

That was my father-in-law's favorite example to those who he felt might lose sight of respecting God's power and will. The hushed tone he used when he related this bit of family history and the awe with which he expressed the danger of challenging God was evident in his body language every time he told it.

As mentioned, my *comadre*, Maggie, and I routinely attended Mass. Armando didn't usually accompany her, but Lupe and my children went with me. None of the Zertuches noted our weekly Mass attendance either to criticize or praise it. We weren't treated as goody-two-shoes or any better or any worse. That's what we chose to do, and they respected it without envying or emulating the habit. That in itself was rare, because they always had comments on everything else we or any other member of the family did. We daughters-in-law found out early that it was easier to laugh with them than to try and swim against the current of their playful banter. Still, their joking excluded the subjects of God, faith and Catholicism. Other than that, all other topics were fair game.

Hopefully, this brief detour will give some perspective to our bond with God. It's not a defense, excuse or affirmation of a right versus a wrong way to practice one's faith. It's merely an explanation, presented without judgment, of where God and faith stood with the family.

3

Growing Up in La Familia

Sylvia was five when my daughter, Cynthia, was born. Terri and Sylvia's brother, Gilbert, was born six weeks after Cynthia, and as they grew older, the two younger cousins forged a close relationship. From the time Cynthia became aware of the tradition of choosing escorts for the *quinceañera* parties traditionally given for young girls when they turned fifteen, she'd decided that Gil would fill that role.

Terri, Sylvia and Cindy (no one but me calls her Cynthia) became a trio whenever the families gathered. And we gathered a lot. Every Sunday after Mass, we drove over to my mother-in-law's for breakfast. She made the best flour tortillas in the world, as well as *papitas* (fried potatoes), *queso con chile* (melted cheese with chili) and other Mexican dishes. Everyone knew she didn't have much interest in housekeeping, but she was certainly one of the best cooks and bakers I've ever known. She truly enjoyed cooking for her brood. By the time we arrived at the house after noon Mass on Sundays, her other sons and their families were already there.

Three of Maria and Mathias' six sons were married; the three younger ones, Robert, Henry and Carlos, were teenagers and still in school. Our *compadres* lived merely two doors away from the in-laws; Serjio, his wife, Josie, and their family of three boys and two girls lived in the same town, South San Francisco. We lived at the northernmost edge of the town, a couple of miles away, so we were all in pretty close proximity to the family headquarters on Railroad Avenue. The ritual Sunday mornings at the Zertuche house were loud and full of good food. Multiple conversations went on at the same time, each in high decibels. Not that the raised voices signaled raised tempers; they simply provided a means to be heard over the verbal melee.

When speaking to or with my in-laws, the sons and daughters-in-law spoke Spanish. We always spoke in Spanish in front of Matias, who didn't speak English other than a few words at his job with McLellan's Orchid Farm. Maria was bilingual, having attended school in South City for a few years in the late 1920s when she, her father and three brothers lived here. When jobs became scarce in the early thirties, her father took his family back to his home state of Coahuila, Mexico. Her slightly-accented English remained very good. Our children spoke mostly with her in English. They spoke butchered Spanish to their grandfather, and some of the Spanish words they created were hysterically funny. Other times it was comical to see the expression on his face as one of our kids tried to explain something to him. Ultimately, he'd end up asking his wife, "Maria, *que dice?*" ("Maria, what is he saying?") Today, our kids' speech might be labeled Spanglish. At the time, we called them "*pochos*," meaning a California-born Mexican, when they couldn't converse properly in Spanish.

Terri and Sylvia, as the older cousins, did a fair job of speaking Spanish under their grandparents' roof. At home and in all other places, they spoke English—unless they didn't want something to be understood by a non-Spanish speaking person. My Joe and Cynthia didn't do as well. Both understood what was being said in Spanish, and Joe could fake his way through some phrases. For instance, when he was thirteen, the four of us took a trip to Mexico City and stayed with my father-in-law's relatives. The wife asked Joe how old he was. Joe managed to say, in Spanish, that he was ten and three years old. Cynthia, on the other hand, understands less Spanish and doesn't speak it at all. However, I suspect that both are familiar with some swear words or impolite phrases.

This mixture of English and Spanish was typical among most Mexican families whose heads of household came from the old country.

Other relatives and family friends usually followed the same language pattern. It was quite common to see many of these relatives and friends at my in-laws' on Sundays. They dropped by knowing that they could count on good food and a boisterous good time. All were welcomed and all were invited to eat. Actually, eating was insisted upon.

The kitchen was geared for large family dining. Mando and Serjio had done some remodeling in their mother's kitchen so that it boasted new cabinets, counters and flooring. It was the most important room in the house. A small chromium table with a gray faux-marble top and four matching chairs rested in front of the stove and sink at one end of the room. It served as the main tortilla-making station from which Grandma Maria kneaded the *masa*, pinched off small balls about the size of apricots, and expertly rolled them out into tortillas about the size of a salad plate.

Every region of Mexico seems to have its own tortilla-making style. Some are very large, others about eight inches in diameter. Maria's were smaller than the norm. They were the size common in the north of Mexico—the state of Coahuila, where the Zertuches were from.

With a twist of her wrist, the raw tortillas were tossed onto the pre-heated *comal*, a flat griddle, on the stove behind her. They bubbled up as they cooked, a sign that they'd be light. There would be one quick flip of the tortilla to allow the other side to cook. Then they were placed on a layered stack within a round bowl which was lined with a clean dish towel. Her tortillas were scrumptious!

The little table was also the official bean-cleaning site. Beans were spilled out onto the cleaned tabletop, separated, purged of tiny specks of dirt, and tossed into a special bean pot. They were then rinsed in cold water several times before cooking. In our family, we don't soak the beans. It's our habit to put them on the stove in the morning with some salt and let them simmer for a few hours.

Another custom from her northern Mexican birthplace was to refry the beans whole, without mashing. The first day, the beans were called "*frijoles de la olla*" (beans from the pot) and were eaten straight out of the pot. The following day, they were fried in a little lard without being mashed. The days of ingesting foods cooked in lard are behind us in these enlightened days, but, boy, there isn't anything that compares with beans and potatoes fried in lard or bacon grease!

The kitchen was a long room. It could have easily been split in half with each half still ample enough to be considered an average-sized kitchen. A larger, round table that seated twelve comfortably rested at the opposite end of the kitchen from the sink and stove. Stacks of boxes were piled in one corner. They held sewing patterns, recipes from ladies magazines, yarns, embroidery thread and other important items that Maria needed at the ready. A back door opened to a small storeroom used as a pantry. From there, a door led to a small porch with five steps down to an enormous yard. The kitchen was Maria's favorite room. It was where she could always be found, and it exuded aromas that today rarely perfume the air.

The house was old, but the Zertuche boys had remodeled, painted, replaced dry rot, and covered the outside with vinyl siding. Matias took great pride in being a homeowner, especially since his sons maintained it. The roof over the front porch was a recurring nuisance and leaked every rainy season. No matter what they did to fix it, it refused to remain fixed. It was patched, ripped off and replaced. Yet it still leaked. Finally, they resorted to calling in a roofing contractor, and for a few years it held up before falling back into its old tendency. It was not uncommon to see buckets or pans on the enclosed front porch when it rained. But Maria loved her very first and only house and filled it with the cooking smells that tantalized and drew in her family.

Addressing each other politely and correctly is a big deal in our families. In Spanish, *mi hija* means "my daughter." *Mija* is a derivative of that term, and *mijita* is the diminutive, endearing form that we all used with our daughters, nieces and young female relatives. Likewise, *mi hijo* means my son; *mijo* is a corruption of that, and *mijito* is the same endearing form used for our young boys. So in our family, *mija* and *mijo* are terms used for all our children, even with our friends' children. For instance, my dear friend, Rosina, calls our children *mijo* and *mija,* and we reciprocate. During their upbringing, our children had scads of *tios* and *tias,* and we had a like number of *mijos* and *mijas*. So, for us to call our nieces and nephews *mijo* and *mija* was a natural, everyday occurrence in most Mexican families.

When Lupe and I walked into my mother-in-law's house, the children immediately greeted us with, "Hi, *tio* or *tia*," meaning uncle and aunt. When Sylvia greeted us, she said, "Hi, *nino, nina*." My response to her was, "Hi, *mijita*," issued with a special tone that implied our unique closeness. This might seem inconsequential to some, but to us, it's important. I believe that this special way of greeting contributes a sense of warmth, security and emotional stability for our children, and it's a custom that also holds true with my own side of the family.

Our family gatherings at the in-laws' were such an integral part of our lives and of our children's upbringing that Sundays automatically meant breakfast at Grandma's. After the children ate, they were usually shooed onto the front porch or out to the back yard to play. Once Terri and Sylvia got older, they were allowed to go home, a couple of doors down, and play games or watch television, away from the rowdy boy cousins.

Invariably, they dragged Cindy along. Their favorite name for her was "the brat." While Terri made fun of how Cindy's outfits always matched down to the hair ribbons or barrettes, she still took her younger cousin under her wing and treated her as a little sister, as did Sylvia. Cindy loved spending time with her two older cousins, and that never changed. Watching the trio interact was great fun. Even though the three cousins had distinctive features, they looked like sisters mainly because they acted like sisters.

Cynthia definitely favors her father's family. She has the same high forehead of her great-grandmother, dark eyes, a sparkling smile and outgoing disposition. Unlike Sylvia's and mine, her hair is naturally curly. Sylvia's locks were a dark, glossy shade of chocolate, whereas mine were a medium brown with chestnut highlights. Many a time, as Sylvia approached and passed her teenage years, we commiserated over possessing such unmanageable hair.

"Why can't it be just a little bit curly? Wavy even," Sylvia would complain as she brushed her tresses.

"I know what you mean, *mija*. At least straight hair is in with your generation. You're right in style."

"Ay, *nina*," she'd say with a wide smile. I heard that comment a lot. Its meaning is very similar to the Irish saying of, "Oh, go on with ye now."

About the time Terri and Sylvia became teenagers, their dad bought a ski boat. His cousin, Manuel, also had one, and both families started camping at Lake Turlock Campgrounds, a few miles south of Don Pedro Dam Lake, near Modesto. Since the dam and reservoir were fairly new in the seventies, the campground trees planted along its shores were young and afforded little shade. As a result, we camped at the more mature and grassy Lake Turlock Campground and drove the short distance to Don Pedro Lake for boating and water skiing.

Don Pedro Dam Lake is the largest man-made lake in California. I happened to have worked for the construction company that built the dam, the Guy F. Atkinson Company of South San Francisco, now out of business. It played a major role in creating the vast network of California dams erected to harness the water from the Sierras in order to green the San Joaquin and Central Valleys. Reservoirs provide popular boating, fishing and camping recreation facilities. But times have changed with concerns for the environment, and dams are no longer being constructed.

Don Pedro Dam boasts one of the largest shorelines of any man-made body of water in the state. The reservoir itself is an enormous, sapphire-blue lake aglitter with white sequined patches created by the brilliant sunlight spotlighting its surface. This vast area shimmers at the foot of the mother lode country near Sonora. The surrounding amber hills illustrate why California is called the Golden State. Most of the year the hills are yellow with tall grasses. A golden hue lines the two-lane highway, broken only by remnants of stone boundaries left by Chinese laborers of the Gold Rush era. Majestic hundred-year-old oaks afford cows little shade.

The three-hour drive to the lake made it handy for weekend visits, and we went as often as we could. Gradually, other members of the family started camping, as well as several close friends and their children. Lupe and I also bought a seventeen-foot ski boat, which made three boats available for water-skiing.

As more relatives, friends and their families swelled our ranks, we eventually required four or five campsite reservations in order to accommodate everyone. We started going up on three-day weekends and for a whole week twice each summer. Some went more often than others. On one occasion, I counted 14 adults and 19 children, most of whom were related. All our kids learned to water-ski, and more importantly, to interact with one another in a family environment.

After dinner, the girls and boys usually separated to do their own thing, mainly strolling around the camp park with their portable radios. By this time, Terri and Sylvia were young teenagers, as were the daughters of a couple of other family friends. Cindy was still the youngest girl cousin at camp, but compatible with the older girls. Everyone enjoyed each other's company.

My son Joe's features favored mine to the point that it was not uncommon for people to ask him if he was my son without knowing whom he belonged to. I doubt that he appreciated the comparison. In age, he was about in the middle of the boy cousins and considered one of the funniest. His antics cracked them up.

After dinner, the adults gathered around the campfire. Lupe and Andres, a close family friend, would pull out their guitars and we would all sing the boleros and ranchera songs that were the Mexican hits of our courting days. One night as we were singing to the guitars, I glanced toward our campsite and saw a burst of light. I bolted out of my aluminum lawn chair and sprinted across the grassy area for about 50 yards to find that Joe had tried to light the camp stove and the corner of the tablecloth had caught fire. By the time I reached the table, several others were behind me, and we easily put out the flames with a couple of strong slaps from dish towels and water from the coffee pot.

"Remember the time when Joey lit up the tablecloth…" was heard for several months afterward.

Sylvia and the other girls kidded the boys about their antics at camp, shaking their heads in disbelief at what was obviously the deficient mental capacity of their brothers. This made the boys clown around even more. Holding contests to see who could burp or fart the loudest was disgusting, in the girls' view, although it did provide plenty of opportunities to make fun of the boys. Despite it all, they got along well while maintaining a certain separateness, perhaps as a defense against contamination.

It was hot at the lake, and the young trees were no protection from the sun. As a result, we spent a lot of time in the water, either skiing or swimming. The boats took turns giving the kids and adults chances to ski, and most got several chances per day. Sylvia was as graceful on water skis as she was on land. I can still see her gliding behind the boat, sprays of rooster tails fanning out in her wake. After cruising the expansive lake, when she was ready to come in she'd release her grip from the rope, coast in with hands raised high, and gradually glide towards shore. At about three feet from the lake's edge, the skis stopped and her body tipped gracefully into the water. It often reminded me of one of Esther Williams' movie scenes.

Even on land, Sylvia had a special gait, striding with arms held slightly out, hands artfully positioned, almost as if she were a model walking down a New York City fashion runway. She looked down at her feet as she started off, as if to check that they had a proper lead, then lifted her head high and floated to her destination. Both Terri and Cindy had her walk down pat and were quick to imitate it whenever they were making fun of her. Sylvia, too, was adept at imitating her sister and cousin, so no one ever remained an unscathed target for long.

Heaven only knows what other things they laughed at in the separate tent reserved for the girls. Sometimes they bunched up in one of the truck camper shells, girl cousins and female friends, to sleep, and the ensuing giggling caused enough movement to rock the truck. More than one portable radio played favorite songs. I sometimes suspected that the radios might have been a camouflage technique to hinder eavesdropping.

Sylvia was one of the most opinionated in the pack. She was frank in her assessments, gentle in their delivery and unwavering in her opinions. The world was quite simple. There was good and bad, sad and happy, dumb and smart. Make your choice and live with it was her philosophy.

"I'm sorry, *nina*, but I have no sympathy for him (or her). He knew what he was doing, what the consequences would be and did it anyway. So…" That was her stock comment about anyone she felt had acted foolishly, whether it was a notorious movie star, her brother, her cousins or whoever. When she felt Terri or Cindy was out of line, they got a bit more leeway. Nonetheless, it was accompanied with an earnestly-delivered critique. The duo almost knew what was coming. They listened, ignored it and carried on. I can still see them tolerantly and good-naturedly rolling their eyes at one of Sylvia's spiels.

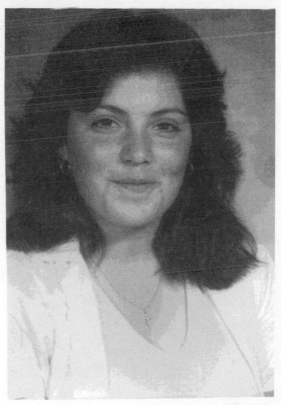

Sylvia M. Zertuche, sophomore year school photo, 1979. Her mouth is closed because she was wearing braces and didn't want them to show.

At fifteen, Sylvia had her *quinceañera*, the equivalent of a debutant party in our Mexican culture. It was held at the Woman's Club in South City, a small hall on Grand Avenue with a large dance floor, kitchen and dining area. Joe was one of the fifteen escorts, but Cindy, at ten years of age, was too young to participate in the entourage that made up the fourteen couples. The *quinceañera* celebrant and her escort provided the symbolic fifteenth pair. Sylvia wore a long pink formal, but would have been more comfortable in the shorts or sweat suits she loved to wear. The boys wore tuxedos.

After the special Mass, we congregated at the Woman's Club, where the live band played the customary opening waltz as her *nino* whisked her around the dance floor. At a certain interval, the rest of her party of fourteen teenage couples joined them in waltzing (which took weeks of practice). We swelled our chests with pride to see our children looking so beautiful, handsome and chic.

I remember her telling me prior to the party, "Oh, *nina*, I'm so nervous."

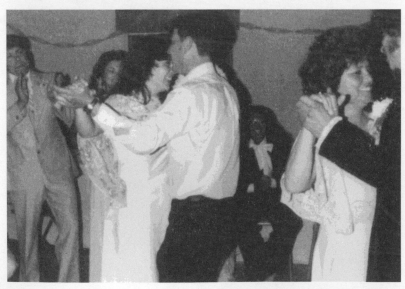

Sylvia's quinceañera party at the South San Francisco Woman's Club, June 1979. From right to left: Mom Maggie with white corsage, Dad Armando in white shirt dancing with Sylvia, Joe, Sr. in beige suit, and Bel's partial face next to him.

"Don't be nervous, *mija*. Everyone here is family or friends. Tell me, who don't you know? You've been to lots of them yourself. It'll turn out fine. Don't worry, we've got everything covered."

Her favorite reply to me was always, "Ay, *nina*," as she smiled and shook her head.

As the evening wore on, the nervousness disappeared. The dances of the young ranged from a Latin beat to rock and roll, and the latest popular gyrations were performed with great gusto. We adults were lucky to sneak in a bolero or a cha-cha occasionally. Everyone stepped to the music in their own fashion. Sylvia was in her element on the dance floor. Never a flashy swiveler, she was cool and smooth, moving totally engrossed in the music. Hers was defined foot movement with suave gestures that never missed a beat and contained just the right, occasional signature touch to show that she was really into the rhythm. That night, I don't think she missed a dance, unless it was one of our old fogey ones.

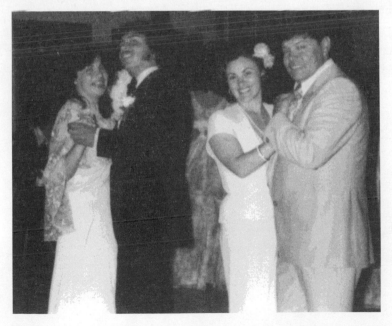

Sylvia's quinceañera party, June 1979. Sylvia dancing with cousin Jim Zertuche. Whoops! Braces are showing. Tios and godparents Bel and Joe, Sr. join in the traditional first waltz.

Mando and Maggie were, of course, very proud of their daughter and reveled in the party. Their sparkle and easy laughter added to any gathering. But on this night, they were at their best. Maggie's petite, five-foot-two frame showed off her formal gown as she and Mando syncopated to almost every dance. Her gorgeous green eyes, pert nose and dynamite smile complemented her handsome husband. Mando, about five foot ten inches, reminded me of Dean Martin with his dark hair, fair skin, and fabulous smile. They were perfectly matched in looks, bubbly personalities and popularity. I don't know of anyone who had more fun at a party than those two.

The morning after the party, Sylvia was at her grandparents' house. As usual, the whole family had congregated for breakfast, and the main topic of conversation consisted of rehashing the previous evening—it would provide conversation fodder for weeks.

"*Mija*, how are you feeling this morning? Tired?" I gave her a big hug as she sat at the big table in her favorite outfit, shorts and a t-shirt. She stood and took her dish to the sink, where Terri was stuck washing dishes.

"Ay, *nina*. I'm soooo tired. I'm going home now to take a nap as soon as I help Teti finish up." She let a huge yawn escape.

"That's okay, *mija*, you go on, we'll finish up," Maggie said as she replaced Terri. I grabbed another dish towel to help my *comadre*. I knew she had to be as tired as I was. We'd closed up the hall after all the guests left and hadn't gotten much sleep.

"Well, come on, brat. Let's go," Terri called to Cindy.

"Wait. Let me grab a few *papitas* and a tortilla." Cindy rushed to gather her breakfast-on-the-run.

"Don't forget the beans." Terri let out her famous, high-pitched cackle because she knew her cousin couldn't stand beans. She's been threatened by the family to have her Mexican-American status taken away for that deficiency.

Sylvia, too tired to expend energy on repartee, began saying her goodbyes, which, in this family, took a while by the time all the *tias* and *tios* were covered. She saved me for last. With a kiss and prolonged hug, she said, "*Nina*, thank you so much for helping out last night. It was really nice."

"Did you have a good time, *mija*?" When she nodded, I added, "Well, then it was well worth it. I'm glad you liked it. Go rest, don't let the gossiping keep you awake." I pointed towards Terri and my daughter.

She delivered the same thanks and acknowledgment to her *nino*, yelled at Terri and Cindy that she couldn't wait any longer, and pranced out the front door. The two others quickly followed. Since Sylvia was such a good sleeper, she'd nap while the other two sat on her bed and talked a mile a minute about the *quinceañera*, especially about the people, both adults and kids, and who'd been present. It wasn't called gossip; it was "remembering."

"Did you see him give her the eye?" Terri started Cindy's education on remembering. She and Terri still continue these conversations long distance.

A major part of any party's fun was always the aftermath, going over every detail, faux pas, nuance, look and comment. Terri and Cindy threw themselves into the task. Sylvia stirred from her nap occasionally to add her two cents, correct a statement, disagree with a comment or scold the other two for their uncharitable remarks, although scolding while laughing is hardly effective.

4

Kidney Failure

Sylvia's passion for dogs came to full bloom with Smokey, the family's Alaskan husky that she doted on for most of her teen years. They were inseparable. At camp, she was usually the one with his leash in her hand, walking him around or securing him and making sure water and food dishes were properly filled. He was the first to get a morning greeting rub and the last one to get a goodnight hug. Certainly she preferred his company to that of many people.

Unfortunately, Smokey brings out guilt for me, and I'll always regret the unwitting tactlessness that might have marred my relationship with Sylvia. During a quiet, uneventful time (in a normally hectic life), our *compadres* told us one night while we were over at their house for coffee that, for some reason I can't recall, Smokey had to be put down. There was definitely no other alternative, according to the vet. The anguish on their faces was evident because they'd enjoyed Smokey for many years. He was a family member, and the time for doing the humane thing for a pet is never easy. Sadly, they'd accepted the vet's judgment.

This conversation took place on a weeknight. The following weekend, after learning of Smokey's death at my mother-in-law's, we went over to our *compadres'* house again. The first person I saw when entering the house was Terri, and I offered my sympathy on the loss of their dog. She stared at me.

"What, *tía*? He ran away. We've been looking for him and hope to find him… what do you mean?" She glanced from mother to father.

Both looked sheepish, and I realized how firmly I'd stuck my foot into my mouth. It had never occurred to me that our *compadres* hadn't told the kids the truth. Apparently, they'd decided to soften his disappearance with a little white lie. I was mortified at my remarks and tried to make up for my mistake.

"Oh, that's what I meant, *mija*. I'm sorry he's gone. That's what I meant. He may show up sometime when you least expect it, you never know. There's lots of stories where dogs make it back to their homes after being lost for a long time…"

Terri was too sharp to be taken in. Turning to her mom, she demanded, "What really happened to him, Mama?"

Maggie and Mando tried their best to explain the situation to Terri and came clean. "We didn't want to tell you kids, especially Sylvia. But we had to do it. The vet said it was the humane thing to do. You know, *mija*, that we wouldn't have done it if there'd been any other way."

Maggie had a painful look on her face. Mando's familiar smile was gone. Terri's face reflected terrible shock. She ran upstairs to her room, slamming the door behind her. Gilbert had wandered into the room quietly without being noticed. He simply bowed his head and said nothing before retreating back to his bedroom. I felt horrible and wished the floor would open up to swallow me whole.

"*Comadre*, I'm so sorry. I never dreamt that they didn't know about it. I just never would have said anything if I'd known. I'm so sorry…"

They were extremely gracious about it. "Oh, don't worry, *comadre*. It's all right. We thought it'd be better the other way. I guess they were bound to find out sooner or later," Mando said.

Maggie chimed in, "It's all right, don't worry. It'll be fine." Then sighing, she added, "Nothing can bring him back. It'll be okay with time, has to be."

It sounded like she was trying to convince herself rather than me. Sylvia immediately came into my mind, and I dreaded the moment she heard the truth. The incident bothered me for days, and I kept rehearsing in my mind what I'd say to Sylvia the next time we met.

As it happened, a few days later, the *compadres* were at our house on a weekend. As usual, we were chatting and laughing over coffee. Suddenly, Sylvia burst in through the unlocked front door. By this time, she was seventeen and had her license, so she'd taken the family jeep to drive over. Her face was white and distorted with anguish. The four of us were sitting in the dining room, immediately visible as the door flew open.

"Tell me the truth, Mama. What happened to Smokey? Why did you tell me that he'd run away?" She was leaning against the wall, sobbing out her words. Closing her eyes, she slowly slid down to the floor and sat in a crumpled heap. Tears ran.

The pain on my *compadre*'s and *comadre*'s faces matched my own. Mando tried to explain, "*Mija... mija,* we didn't have a choice..."

Maggie rose to go over to Sylvia. Kneeling to put her arm around her, she murmured Terri's childhood name for her sister. "Chiva, *mija,* shhhh, it's okay. This is why we couldn't bring ourselves to tell you. We knew how devastating it would be for you. *Mija,* please... try to understand."

I couldn't tell if Sylvia could hear her. I got up from my chair to approach the two when Sylvia stood up and paced furiously around the dining room table. "You should have told me! You should have told me! Here I've been looking out my window, driving around, hoping to catch sight of him, and for what? For nothing! Nothing! He's gone. Dead! And you hid it from me!" I'd never seen Sylvia so upset or felt so helpless.

Turning to me, she accused, "And you, *nina!* You knew and didn't tell me. How could you..." Her voice choked into silence. She sat down and cradled her face in her arms. Nothing could make the situation better. She lifted her head, eyes swollen, and ran out as abruptly as she'd whirled in, leaving the air thick with her anguish.

"God, *comadre.* I'm so very sorry. I wish I'd known..." For me to go on would have been pointless.

Remaining compassionate while in her own torment, she said, "Oh, don't worry, *comadre*. Maybe we should've been honest from the beginning. But this is the very thing we wanted to avoid. We knew she'd take it hard." Maggie looked exhausted.

Mando said nothing, just sat and tugged at his hair, a nervous habit of his. They rose to go home and face what needed to be endured and appeased. With time, the crisis receded, but the subject of Smokey's absence was never mentioned in Sylvia's presence. Everyone was mindful of this taboo, young and old alike. It took a long time for me to get over my blunder. Yet Sylvia never demonstrated any bitterness toward me. She and my *compadres* were more forgiving to me that I was to myself.

How quickly the time arrived for Sylvia's high school graduation! One Sunday in early May, while making our usual grandparents visit, she pulled out her graduation picture from a large envelope. It was an eight-by-ten photo personally inscribed to her *ninos*. As I sat at the big table, coffee mug in hand, I marveled at the beautiful young woman in the formal pose of a senior who'd morphed into this dark-haired beauty. Where were the faded shorts, the sweat suits? Who was this glamour puss beaming at me? My little godchild was now a beautiful young woman. "Watch out, world," I proudly thought.

"So, what do you think you want to do, *mija*? Go to college?" I asked.

"Umm, maybe I'll go to community college, get my general ed requirements out of the way. First I'll look for a part-time job and then try to fit my schedule around it." She wrinkled up her pert nose. "Oh, I'm not sure, *nina*. Right now I have to make sure I pass my finals. They're next week."

"You'll pass, *mija*, just be sure you study. When you're ready, let's sit down and talk about your plans. There's a lot out there for you, *mija*." We'd had conversations before about continuing her education, and she knew how strongly I felt that it was the key to a good future for her. I felt confident that whatever she decided she wanted to do or be was doable. Once she made up her mind, she would focus.

"Okay, *nina*. But, what I'm really looking forward to is camping all summer and water skiing." Her eyes danced.

"I call it sitting in the dirt, *mija*. But I know you kids love it, and it's fun, despite all the work. I get a big kick out of making café amore for everyone at night." My cousin, who was in fine foods distribution to restaurants in San Francisco and the Peninsula, kept me stocked with restaurant-sized cans of café amore, which is a powdered coffee, milk and chocolate mixture—similar to a rich mocha. The adults drank their café amore with brandy; the kids had it straight. And they all clamored for it, not letting me go one night without making it.

"We love it, too, *nina*. Everything always seems wonderful at camp, doesn't it." It was a statement, not a question.

Sylvia needed a nap, and Terri and Cindy followed her home, their refuge from the adults who were congregated around the huge table. As usual, their departure was slowed by the number of goodbyes and hugs issued to all the *tias* and *tios*, just in case some of us left before they returned.

"Come on, slowpoke," Terri called to Cindy. "She'll be asleep before we get there if you don't hurry. Boy, that girl can sleep." Obviously, something of importance had to be discussed.

The following week, Sylvia wasn't at her grandmother's on Sunday morning. "She's not feeling well, *comadre*. I think she's got the flu," Maggie said.

After eating, I walked over to Sylvia's house, but not before cautioning Cynthia, "*Mija*, you stay here, just in case it's catchy."

"Oh, Mom, I'll stay downstairs with Terri. I won't go upstairs."

Cynthia ran up the front stairs before me, calling out for Terri. "Shhh, *mija*," I admonished. "Sylvia might be asleep."

"Mom, that girl could sleep through a hurricane. Nothing wakes her up except her own snoring."

Terri was plopped on the living room floor in front of the television set, which was turned down low.

"Hi, brat." That was it, no teasing about her cousin's outfit, no sarcasm.

31

"Hi, *mija*," I whispered. "How's Chiva?"

Terri got up to give me a kiss and hug. "She's asleep, *tia*. She's been sleeping a lot lately. Doesn't feel good. We think it's the flu." She returned to her place on the rug, leaving room for Cynthia to sit down beside her. Terri appeared distracted and not in a mood for banter this morning, and instinctively, Cynthia knew to back off. For a few moments I watched whatever was on the screen without really seeing it, mentally debating whether to go upstairs or not. Ultimately, I decided not to.

"I'll let her sleep, *mija*. When she wakes up, tell her I was here asking about her, okay?"

"Sure, *tia*." Terri didn't take her eyes off the set.

Tousling Cynthia's hair, I said, "*Mija*, we'll be going in about an hour, so come back when the next program is over, okay?" Cynthia nodded, and I walked slowly back to my in-laws', puzzled about Sylvia's getting the flu in early May. She hadn't looked peaked the last time we talked. I quashed a nagging uneasiness that almost frightened me. I knew I'd be calling my *comadre* in a couple of days to check up on Sylvia.

The following Sunday, Sylvia was still feeling under the weather. I asked my *comadre*, "Has she seen the doctor?"

"Yes, *comadre*, I took her to Kaiser and they said to give it another week or so." She shrugged her shoulders. Since we were at our in-laws', we were speaking in Spanish.

"Is she awake at all? Would it be all right to go over?"

"She sleeps a lot, and I think it best that she get all the rest she can. I do wake her up to make her drink liquids. You know her, she likes her water. But I can't get her to drink any juice or teas."

Maggie collected a few dirty plates and headed for the sink. I grabbed the remaining ones, deposited them on the counter and took the sponge to wipe off the plastic tablecloth. Lupe, *compadre*, Serjio and Matias were in the living room watching the San Francisco Giants play baseball. Half of the kids were on the porch and the others were out in front playing since it was such a nice day.

"Are you taking her back to Kaiser?" I asked.

"I'm going to call for an appointment tomorrow, *comadre*."

"Well, don't let them give you the runaround. Insist that she get in. This is too weird, something's…" I trailed off, realizing that my advice was unnecessary. Other thoughts remained better left unsaid. The pensive look on Maggie's face as she swirled the dishrag in hot, soapy water told me that she was as apprehensive as I was about Sylvia's condition.

Later that week, Sylvia was hospitalized.

"Kidney failure!" I shouted in Spanish. "Are you sure, *suegra*?" (mother-in-law)

"That's what Armando told me. She's at Kaiser. He told me to let you know. He just came by to get a quick bite and he's on his way back to the hospital now. I told him to send me Maggie. I'm sure she hasn't eaten yet."

Comfort revolved around being fed, and that was Maria's best expression of support. She'd cook all day and night if she thought it would help.

We said our goodbyes and hung up. I couldn't believe it. I stood by the phone, stunned. There had to be some mistake. "I'll go and get the straight story firsthand," I told myself. "Maybe it's just an infection or something…"

I hurried to finish clearing up the kitchen. It was after dinner, and the kids were sitting at the kitchen table doing their homework. They had heard my conversation and looked up, waiting for an explanation. "I don't know yet, but I'm going over to Kaiser to see your *tios*. Don't worry now. Finish up and you can watch television before your showers, okay?"

Lupe was downstairs in the family room relaxing in his recliner, half watching television and half finishing the paper. I hurried down to repeat the news his mother had just relayed. His forehead wrinkled. "What? Are you sure?"

A lot of people, my grandmother included, thought he looked like Robert Wagner, and I could see the resemblance. He had the same dazzling, trademark smile typical in his family, brown eyes, and a serious nature that was quiet without being sullen. At the moment, he was puzzled, and I assured him, "That's what she said. I want to go over to

Kaiser and see the *compadres*. I think Maggie might still be there. Will you make sure the kids take their showers and get to bed by nine?"

He nodded. "But you'll be back by then, won't you?" I rarely went out at night without him, and I could see he was slightly uncomfortable about it now. Under the circumstances, he held back any reservations and nodded agreement that I should go.

"I hope so, but just in case, that's all."

5

Terri, Sylvia's First Kidney Donor

In South City, Kaiser Hospital is on El Camino Real, about a mile and a half from our house, so it didn't take me long to get there. Our usual summer morning and evening fog was present. Like clockwork, about six in the evening, it furls over the San Bruno mountain range from the Pacific Ocean, slowly descending to envelop the town and dampen the roads in its wanderings. It shimmers under the streetlights, veiling the streets in an ethereal luminescence. I've always loved fog. But tonight it had an eeriness about it that clutched at my heart. Why was I so frightened?

As the mist wrapped around the car, I knew God was just as present and begged for His help. From my parochial school education, I remembered that everyone has a cross to bear and that God gives one the strength to bear it. No one is given more than he or she can endure, so we're told. But I didn't want to have to be strong, didn't want to be tested. I froze my mind, forbidding it to think beyond selecting the right parking space.

At the hospital, I headed for the information counter to get Sylvia's room number. The corridors seemed endless as the staccato beat of my heels ricocheted in my ears. When I finally reached the right room, I was stopped cold by the prevailing silence. My *compadres* sat in the sterile, private room without exchanging a word. He was staring at the floor, and she was gazing out the window, the meager view consisting of gray mist.

Maggie offered me no smile; neither did Mando. Sylvia lay sleeping under a light coverlet, an IV jutting from her wrist. The soft, buzzing sound of her snore resonated against the stark walls.

"Hi *comadre*, *compadre*," I whispered. "*Que pasa?*"

With a heaviness mixed with disbelief, he recounted what he'd been told by the doctors. In Spanish, he said, "One of her kidneys has failed. They don't know why, it's just gone. She's pretty sick, *comadre*." Even as he spoke, it was without conviction that the words he was quoting by rote could possibly be true. But they were.

I turned toward Maggie to say something, but was interrupted by the sound of approaching steps. A woman doctor, file grasped against her chest, entered the room. Dr. Dolislager was tall, which always impresses me because I'm only five feet, one inch, and I envy women who are graced with greater height. Her light brown hair was cut fashionably short, and her hazel eyes were filled with concern as she spoke. I knew from previous conversations with Maggie that Dr. Dolislager was Sylvia's pediatrician and would be her primary doctor at Kaiser until Sylvia turned eighteen, which was an event almost upon us.

"Mr. and Mrs. Zertuche." She nodded a hello and remained standing as she leaned against the inside door jamb.

Sylvia awoke, stirred, saw me and sleepily said, "Hi, *nina*." Then, noticing the doctor, she greeted her also.

"Hi there, Sylvia. It's Dr. Dolislager. How are you feeling today?"

"I'm so sleepy, doctor. Otherwise, I feel okay, just tired."

The doctor turned to Maggie and Mando, and her soft voice took on a businesslike tone. "I've consulted with a nephrologist at the University of San Francisco Medical Center. We consult with them on these matters since they specialize in this type of thing. Dr. Oscar Salvatierra is an expert in this field, and it's his opinion, after reviewing the file, that Sylvia's kidneys are failing. One is totally gone and the other is at sixty percent and is dropping further." She paused to see if we were taking it all in.

Maggie and Mando displayed frozen expressions. My eyes rested on Sylvia, observing her take on the diagnosis. She'd definitely heard every word, but didn't flinch. It took all my willpower to refrain from doing so.

"What's a nephrologist?" I asked.

"That's a kidney specialist," she answered me without taking her eyes off Maggie and Mando.

Maggie frowned and straightened up in her chair. "But why? Why have they failed? What happened?"

"That's what we're not so sure about. Is she on any medication?" Dr. Dolislager queried.

"No. She took aspirin for her headaches when she had the flu, or what we thought was the flu, that's all," Maggie said.

The doctor turned to Sylvia. "Have you been dieting? Maybe taken some diet pills, drugs of any kind?"

"No," Sylvia said almost defensively. "Nothing like that. I haven't taken any kind of pills."

"My daughter doesn't take anything she's not supposed to," Mando said a little defensively.

"I'm just trying to see if we can identify the cause, Mr. Zertuche, that's all. Sometimes acute kidney failure is genetic, a hereditary flaw that's inexplicable." Her tone was soothing. "In any event, we'd like to send Sylvia to Stanford Hospital to be checked out by their nephrology department. When we have those results, we can compare them with UCSF's and go from there."

Maggie's eyes widened. Mando spoke. "We'll do anything we need to do. How soon can she be seen at Stanford?"

Dr. Dolislager became more animated, as if she'd expected confrontation and was pleased that it hadn't materialized. Looking directly at Sylvia, who remained quiet and calm, she said, "Well, first we'll have to stabilize you as much as we can, Sylvia. There's a possibility you'll have to go on dialysis."

Before the doctor could go on, Sylvia promptly asked, "What's dial…"

Dr. Dolislager explained. "Since your kidneys can't filter the toxins in your system, we use a machine that acts like an artificial kidney and cleanses your blood. A shunt is placed in your wrist, similar to an IV, so that we can connect you to the machine easily. It draws out your blood on one side, gets rid of the impurities in it and replaces it with the cleansed blood. We'll show you how it works. Lots of people have to use this on a regular basis, Sylvia. It's routine with patients that have kidney failure. At this point, we don't know how often you'll have to do it. I'm just telling you this so that you know what to expect. We also have to get you some medications. We're going to do everything we can to try and save what remains of your good kidney, Sylvia. You can believe that."

She turned to Maggie and Mando and answered his question. "Give us a couple of days to figure out her medications, stabilize her and then we'll send her down to Stanford. In the meantime, we're going to do some more testing in the next day or two to see if we can get at the bottom of this. But, more importantly than that, we need to arrest the failure if we can, and get Sylvia what she needs to get better. After we get the results back from Stanford, several of us will consult again and maybe have a better grasp of the situation."

Mando's face tightened in anguish. His unconscious habit of tugging at his hair was in play. "But why? Why did this happen? What caused it? She was okay a couple of weeks ago. I just don't understand. We were told she might have the flu, then hepatitis…" He drifted off, letting his words dangle in midair.

"We don't really know in Sylvia's case. We may never know. Though whatever the cause, Mr. Zertuche, I think what we need to do is concentrate on arresting further deterioration of the good kidney and get her on the proper meds." She stopped talking. We continued to look at her, as if by staring we'd extract some little scrap of good news or encouragement.

Sylvia broke the silence and very soberly said, "Thank you, doctor."

"You're welcome." Dr. Dolislager approached the bed and touched Sylvia's leg. "You're a brave girl, Sylvia. I'll be seeing you every day and expect you to let me know everything that's going on with you. The more we know, the more we can help. Okay?"

Sylvia's lips quivered slightly as she shut her eyes and nodded. Tears slid onto her pillow. Dr. Dolislager looked over to the *compadres*, paused a few seconds to see if there were any more questions, and when there were none, prepared to walk out of the room. Before leaving, she glanced at me. My throat was dry, my mind stifled, wanting to reject her assessment. Her words, final and irreversible, screamed for denial. But logic forced its truth on us, numbing us. Sensing the depth of our shock, Dr. Dolislager turned and left, perhaps as weighted as we.

It was so hard to move. Maggie and Mando were quite still. I waited for one of them to make the first move, utter the first word.

"*Mija*, you're going to be all right, you'll see. I like her, don't you? She seems like she really knows what she's doing." Maggie sat on the bed. Mando moved to the foot of the bed and patted Sylvia's thigh lovingly, unable to speak.

Sylvia cried softly for a few moments, and Maggie leaned over and enfolded her in her arms, kissing her cheek and whispering muffled, comforting words. Within a minute or two, Sylvia released a great sigh, turned her head and fell asleep again.

I couldn't move. Why her? Why my Sylvia? Was this real? Deep inside, panic grew because I didn't understand what was happening. I was afraid for where this would lead. Nothing made sense. In this confused state, I didn't even have the presence of mind to pray, although I'd make up for it later.

My *compadres* looked at each other, anxiety in their eyes. Our eyes fell on Sylvia and filled with tears. Tears, resolve and resignation would accompany all of us in the next few weeks.

The tests at Stanford Medical Center in Palo Alto were performed and appraised by Kaiser doctors, who shared the results with UCSF's nephrology department. The *compadres* were shuttled between Kaiser in South City and the UCSF Medical Center on Parnassus Street in the city. It was determined that UCSF would take charge of Sylvia's case. She was released from Kaiser, given several medications and felt well enough to graduate with her class in June, much to our joy and her satisfaction. The possibility of being unable to attend her graduation had really bothered her. Once she found out that she'd be at the ceremony, her spirits were boosted.

During that time, I think we all applied a veneer of normalcy for the sake of our children and ourselves. It might have been an attempt to prop one another up, to keep one foot in front of the other in order not to disturb the symmetry of our lives or frighten the children. To all appearances we carried on with our routines. However, what we hid, what didn't show, gnawed at us day and night. It was the last thing we thought of before going to bed, the first thing upon waking, and what seeped through our thoughts at different times during the day. We adults, who were supposed to be the protectors of our children, were stymied, and it sickened us. That my *compadres* managed to save their sanity was astonishing.

Laughter still rang out in Maria's kitchen at Sunday breakfasts. We continued going to parties and dances at the Morelos Hall. Camping and water skiing still went on at the lake. But foremost in everyone's heart and mind was the fact that our Sylvia's life was endangered. It was like a neon sign flashing within to color our everyday outlook on the world, and nothing blocked it out. Our only hope was the constant petition on our lips to Our Father, the supreme parent. Like pesky children, we pleaded for His intervention while knowing that we could do little else.

Encouragement from family and friends embraced Sylvia, and for a while it seemed like she was getting better. However, Terri, who was the closest to her and experienced every peak and valley with her sister, noticed that Sylvia was more forgetful and sleepy. The doctors said it was a side effect of the medications. All of us noticed that she tired easily. This lethargy, such a contrast to the old Sylvia, came and ebbed. Every day brought something new, sometimes heartening, sometimes discouraging.

The most devastating report came shortly after Sylvia's follow-up appointment at UCSF with Drs. Vincente and Salvatierri, noted nephrologists. Routine urine tests showed that her creatinine levels were way up. Creatinine, contained in our urine, is the measure by which kidney function is assessed. Normal levels should be around one. Hers were in the double digits, indicating that both kidneys were not functioning. Both kidneys were gone. With total failure of the second kidney, regular dialysis treatments became mandatory.

Without a doubt, dialysis is a life-saving technique to those with renal failure. In the absence of functioning kidneys, it washes the toxins out of the bloodstream. It's a routine that takes hours; at least it did at that time. The fact that Sylvia was scheduled for dialysis confirmed the gravity of her situation. Sylvia, despite knowing that her life depended upon using the treatment, viewed it as a horrible reminder of her condition. She knew that she was shackled with that regimen until her turn on the organ waiting list materialized. At that time, the average wait was three years.

The family shared in every new development in Sylvia's condition. Updates during coffee klatches at my in-laws' or at Mando and Maggie's kept us informed. My *compadres* also visited Serjio and Josie, sharing the same information with them. A new vocabulary filtered into our conversations: renal failure, creatinine levels, dialysis, Prednisone, nephrology and organ waiting lists. As Mando and Maggie shared the results from doctors' visits and related the information contained in the pamphlets received from UCSF's transplant unit, our knowledge about kidney failure and its possible consequences expanded. What a drastic change from planning the next family party or camping trip.

Sylvia became conspicuously absent from most Sunday gatherings at Grandma Maria's. When she did come over, it was for a brief appearance. Usually in her shorts or sweats, she entered with an attempted cheery hello to everyone. The springy bounce was still evident, though not in full force. It was difficult to camouflage our reactions on how bloated Sylvia's beautiful face had become from the effects of the Prednisone, a steroid required for her survival. Her one-hundred-and-twenty pound frame had ballooned by at least twenty pounds. It was all I could do to look beyond the puffiness to imagine the hidden Sylvia trapped within that swollen body. Even her voice seemed strained. Her face, dulled by the missing sparkle in her eyes, was not that of our old Sylvia.

"Hi, *tia, tio*." Everyone got the ritual peck.

Compassion softened everyone's tongue. Hellos became verbal embraces. The normal teasing that usually ran rampant in the Zertuche headquarters melted away with her entrance.

"*Mija*, how ya doin'?" Serjio asked.

"Fine, *tio*." The standard reply.

"*Mija*, look in the freezer. I bought you your favorite ice cream," Grandpa Matias said in Spanish. Nothing said love in that household as much as feeding you.

Sylvia tucked a long strand of glossy hair behind her ear. "Oh, thank you, Grandpa. I'll have some later." Her simple Spanish pleased him.

Turning to Cindy, she said in English, "Hear that, brat? He bought that ice cream for me. Hands off." The opportunity to tease transformed a faint smile into a familiar grin, and it thrilled us.

"That's all right, Grandma made me *papitas*," Cindy retorted with a smirk.

I awaited my turn as she finished her hellos around the big table and came over to where her grandma, Maggie, Serjio's wife Josie, and I were seated at the smaller work table.

After our special hug, I said, "Hi, *mija*. Terri just left, did you pass her on your way over here? She says you're going to the movies."

"Yeah, Terri wants to go, but she wants to see some crazy science-fiction movie called *ET*. She wanted me to ask you if the brat could come with us, *nina*."

I looked over to my husband, and he nodded consent. I asked Cindy, "*Mija*, you want to go?" which was a very unnecessary question.

Sylvia grabbed a few *papitas* from Cindy's plate even though a bowl on the stove was full of them. "Well, if you want to go, get moving. You know how impatient Terri gets." She spun around, waved her hand and threw out a smile. "Bye, *tios*. Come on, brat."

Cynthia and Sylvia left. A temporary pall hung over the kitchen, each of us with our own thoughts on how Sylvia's physical appearance was being transformed. There was no point in expressing these feelings, so we didn't. Neither did we question Maggie or Mando, because they had shared all they knew about Sylvia's condition, and the absence of more information was too unsettling. Since the second kidney had failed, we knew Sylvia was on the organ waiting list, even though we were totally ignorant of what that really meant. In our naïveté we assumed that her turn would come up soon.

Gradually, the kitchen came back to life. Mundane conversation seeped through the unspoken sentiments so that if a stranger had walked in, they'd have thought that all was normal in the Zertuche household.

Whenever I caught Terri alone, either at her house or her grandma's, I quizzed her about Sylvia. Terri was privy to the situation in a way that neither her parents nor we were. I took advantage of that insider information whenever I could.

"*Mija,*" I asked Terri. "How is she? Any worse, any better?"

"About the same, *tia*. Sometimes she seems all right, but she forgets a lot." Terri's hazel eyes widened as she nodded. "They say it's the medication. We really have to watch her. And touchy, she's so touchy." Terri elongated the word "touchy" to give it emphasis. "She cries easily, and those headaches, she gets those a lot."

It saddened and disquieted me to see the effect Sylvia's illness was having on Terri. She seemed to have aged in a few short weeks. And she'd become more mature than her nineteen years demonstrated weeks before. Gilbert, too, had to be affected in hidden, unspoken ways. There was a worried look on Terri's face that didn't belong on someone that young. As her *tia*, I was frustrated at not being able to offer my niece any meaningful comfort.

No matter how much we tried to conceal it, Sylvia's condition weighed heavily on each of us, knocking the family off its equilibrium. Lapses occurred when friends or relatives had a party. Baptisms, wedding showers, weddings, baby showers, or birthday parties provided occasional distractions. But in the background, the harsh reality that Sylvia was dangerously ill was ever-present and continued to frighten us. Personally, I knew that everyone was praying for Sylvia, but no one ever expressed that private practice. How Maggie and Mando coped defies understanding, yet we knew there was no other choice. The rest of the family tried to be strong for them and supportive. Unfortunately, that did nothing to resolve the problem.

It was late summer when Lupe and I were sitting at Maggie and Mando's kitchen table laughing over coffee about camping incidents or discussing the latest news from one of the other brothers' families. Terri, Cynthia and Gilbert were either watching television in the living room or upstairs talking. Sylvia slept more and had frequent headaches and spent more of her time quietly in her room.

Maggie got up from the table to refill our cups. I directed myself to Mando.

"So, *compadre*. What do the doctors say? How much longer before Sylvia's turn comes up?" He knew I referred to the organ waiting list.

Maggie sat back down and fidgeted with the paper napkin in front of her, folding the corners and unfolding them. Mando's frown said so much. "I ask and ask, *comadre*, but they say she still has to wait. We don't know what to do. She's going to dialysis, doing everything she's supposed to be doing, taking all her pills. I don't know." His hand was in his hair.

"I like her doctors." Maggie spoke without raising her eyes from the table. "Dr. Salvatierri and Dr. Amend are really nice and supposed to be the tops in their field. This week, when we were up at UCSF, Dr. Amend said that it could be a couple of years before they found a kidney for Sylvia." Her lips tightened into a straight line.

"A couple of years!" I couldn't believe my ears. "You can't wait that long. How can you make plans? How can she go on to school if she doesn't feel well? For God's sake! It's been over three months. This is ridiculous!" It was so frustrating. Then I blurted, "*Compadre*, what if we write a letter? I mean, how can Sylvia get on with her life? And you. This must be killing you. I know it's driving me nuts. They need to know how much it's affecting her, your lives and the rest of the family. Something's got to give."

Maggie looked at Mando as he leaned back in his chair, a hint of hope in his voice. "Sure, *comadre*, if you think it'll help."

"It can't hurt. We sure can't just sit around while nothing's happening. *Comadre*, do you have a writing tablet I can use? Maybe one of the kids has some binder paper."

Pen in hand, I asked, "Okay, let me get this straight. What's the name of the department I should send this to? How do you spell the doctors' names?"

"Let me get their cards, *comadre*." Maggie dashed into the bedroom, returning with her purse. "I've got them in my wallet. Here." She slid them over to me to copy. The activity animated us.

We collaborated on the facts to ensure accuracy. I drafted our thoughts, describing how the status of Sylvia's wait for an organ transplant was demoralizing the family. By the time we finished, there were three pages of shorthand notes in front of me. The twenty minutes or so it took to draft the proposed letter had a positive effect on us. It was as if we'd armed ourselves with a weapon to fight this maddening inactivity. A hopeful glow showed on Maggie and Mando's faces when we said goodnight.

"I'll polish this up, type it and bring it over Sunday for you to sign. Are you going up next week, or do you think we should mail it?"

"Let's mail it, *comadre*. Even if we go up, we're not sure who we're going to see." Maggie followed that with, "Thank you, *comadre*. Maybe that'll help."

The letter was typed, it met with their approval, they signed it and off it went. Two weeks went by, then three. On the third Sunday, our *compadres* had left my in-laws' house before we got there, so we walked over to their house after we'd had breakfast. The door was unlocked and we poked our noses in, calling out their names.

Mando was working on remodeling the rear bathroom, and we could hear the loud buzz of some power tool. Maggie walked down the hallway to greet us. We were standing in the living room, waiting for the signal of where to sit—in the living room or the kitchen. The kitchen always won out. When the power tool was turned off, Mando peeked out from the bathroom door when he heard our voices. "Hi, sit down. I'll be there in a minute."

45

"Coffee?" Maggie asked.

"No, *gracias*, *comadre*. We just had plenty. Where's *mija?*" I asked for Sylvia.

"She's upstairs lying down. Another headache."

I went up the stairs, peeked into Sylvia's bedroom and found her asleep. I returned to the kitchen.

"Have you had any reply to the letter yet?" I asked, impatient to get to the reason for our visit.

"Yes, *comadre*, we did," Maggie replied.

By this time, Mando, brushing chalky sheet rock dust from his pants, sat down to join us.

"We did, *comadre*," he said. "They wanted to know if a lawyer had written it." He laughed.

I laughed, too. "So does that mean I can send you a bill?" Their faces looked somewhat relieved, and Lupe and I eagerly leaned forward for whatever news they had.

Maggie took the lead. "Well, they really explained things to us. You know, *comadre*, at first we were so upset about what happened that maybe we didn't pay enough attention to what they were saying about the waiting list. It turns out that there are lots of people waiting for kidneys, thousands. It could be two or three years before Sylvia is eligible. They were explaining that…"

Mando interrupted, "The thing is that she has a good chance of being called within that time if she stays healthy. She's young and is better off than some of the patients waiting their turn. They take the most critical ones first, then it depends on getting a good match. It seems pretty fair to everybody, it's just that there's so many waiting."

The conversation finally reached the bottom line, which was that Sylvia was no further ahead or better off. But we did achieve a better understanding of how the waiting list worked. All the nuances of their conversation with the doctors were repeated and rehashed until I felt I'd gotten a thorough account of their discussions.

It was hard to be satisfied when resolution of the problem seemed no closer. Yet I had the impression that something remained unsaid. I couldn't quite put my finger on it, but I definitely sensed it. I found it difficult to accept the status quo, but concealed my dissatisfaction from them. We ended our visit and went home with a better understanding of the waiting period, but not much else.

Several weeks later, the family received a great surprise. Terri was going to donate her kidney to her sister! The news floored Lupe and me, our kids and the rest of the family. Was this the reason our *compadres* had looked more hopeful a couple of Sundays ago? That gleam of hope I'd detected was named Terri. Had this alternative solution to the waiting list been presented to them by the doctors after my letter had been received? Was the reason they didn't say anything then to make sure Terri was a good match for her sister? Whatever the reason, Sylvia's world had spun upright again, as had ours. She became visibly animated, and her walk showed some of that old bounce again. We were all bouncier and so very grateful to our niece.

Through Terri we felt that our prayers had been answered. She seemed to take the event in stride as we all sat back in admiration. At twenty, this young woman was our champion and her sister's savior. Even Cynthia was impressed to the point of letting Terri win some of their arguments. Joe, his cousins and their friends were equally moved as all of us rejoiced in the anticipation of the transplant surgery. Terri had lifted the worrisome clouds from the family and become our heroine.

However, any attempt to praise her for her generosity met with a dismissive remark. She trivialized it.

"Oh, *tia*, it's nothing. No big deal. I know that Chiva would do the same for me." She wasn't indulging in false modesty. It truly was simply a matter of providing her sister with something she was able to give, and nothing could be more natural. It was as natural as love.

From that time forward, she no longer was the little niece when she walked into the kitchen. She was our brave rescuer, and as such, commanded a deepened respect and esteem. Terri and Sylvia became even closer as they shared the final testing process and walked hand in hand toward the resolution of Sylvia's problem.

6

Sylvia's First Successful Transplant

It was the Sunday prior to Sylvia's and Terri's operations at UCSF Medical Center—Sylvia's as the transplant recipient and Terri's as the kidney donor. The Zertuche kitchen was full of excitement at the expected results of the surgery. If anyone felt a tinge of apprehension at the effect on Terri, it wasn't voiced. We'd all been assured that she'd be fine. She was young and in good health, and the emotional bond shared between the two was a positive aspect that enhanced Terri's standing as a good match. We were optimistic that it would have a successful outcome. For insurance, we offered up prayers. Of late, the votive candle in front of my mother-in-law's statute of the Virgen de Guadalupe was constantly lit.

Repeated queries to Terri asking if she felt nervous were serenely answered with a firm, "No." It was accompanied by a toss of her head and that little pucker of her lips which labeled her a Bernal, Grandmother Maria's side of the family. We couldn't assure her enough of our support and love. It was a time when her name was mentioned reverently.

"So, *mija*. What were the results of the last test? Have they decided which one to take?" I knew that she'd undergone a procedure in which dye was injected into her kidneys to enable the surgeons to view them, evaluate their position and determine which was the best one to extract.

"It went all right, *tia*. I don't know which one they decided on." With a nonchalant shrug of her shoulders, she added, "It really doesn't

49

matter, I don't care." That famous laugh was followed by, "I hope it's the heaviest one so that I'll lose some weight."

Terri, petite at five foot one inch, is neither slender nor chubby. Perhaps full-bodied for her height is more descriptive. She has a pretty face reminiscent of Michelangelo's famous cherubs, complete with curls, full cheeks and rosy complexion. Her wide toothsome smile, inherited from her parents, beams out. Her greenish eyes, like her mother's, light up a room like a dancing sunbeam.

Is there a parent, family member or friend who isn't nervous prior to a loved one's going into surgery? How about when you have two loved ones under the knife? We were no different. I can only guess at what Maggie and Mando felt with both daughters about to undergo major surgery. Yes, it was a life-saving procedure for Sylvia, but it was also a major trauma for Terri. Our comfort was encouraged by the fact that the surgery was taking place at a highly-renowned institution whose transplant unit was considered one of the best in the nation. It helped that they had two of the finest doctors handling Sylvia's case, and that the surgeons performing the nephrectomy procedure were experts in their field.

Most of all, it helped that we had our faith as an anchor. Maggie attended All Souls Church's Spanish Mass as a rule. Having been raised in Mexico, she welcomed hearing the Mass and sermon in Spanish. Lupe and I belonged to St. Veronica's parish, and our children went to that parochial school. We attended Mass as a family every week. Having been educated here in parochial schools, my level of spiritual comfort was fostered by hearing the Mass in Latin and English as it had been in my youth. Even if St. Veronica's had held Mass in Spanish, I would have continued going to the English language services.

My in-laws didn't attend Mass, nor did the rest of the brothers. Not that they didn't believe in God; it just wasn't a habit they'd ever gotten into. Nonetheless, there remained a solid foundation of faith. Every home had a crucifix, a Virgen de Guadalupe statue or picture, and votive candles. The Virgen de Guadalupe is our special Madonna, and it is to her that we pray in hard times. It's a rare Mexican household that doesn't have her image on some wall or shelf.

Before leaving for home from my in-laws' on the Sunday prior to the big surgery, we slipped over to the *compadres'* house. All the occupants were acting normally—watching television, reading the newspaper, sipping coffee—yet the atmosphere was charged. Terri and Sylvia were out.

"They ran over to the drugstore to pick up some toiletries, *comadre*. They should be back soon." Maggie practically sang out the words.

"So, are they all right? Is Terri nervous?" I asked.

Lupe had joined Mando in the living room to watch whatever Forty-Niner football game was on. Joe had remained outside playing with his cousins, including Gilbert. Cynthia sat next to her dad on the sofa, eagerly waiting for her cousins to return.

"They're okay, *comadre*." I could tell she was trying to remain subdued in anticipation of the morning. The overall mood simulated a tea kettle ready to go off. She looked at me, eyes filled with emotions held in check.

"Tomorrow they go in for the standard pre-op tests—you know, EKG, lungs, blood, urine, etc. Sylvia will get a dialysis treatment."

I interrupted to add, "Hopefully, for the last time, *comadre*."

"*Dios primero, comadre*." (The literal translation is "First God," but it means "God willing.")

"Do you know what time surgery is on Tuesday?"

"We'll find out for sure sometime tomorrow. Mando's going to work, but I'll be there all day. He's taking Tuesday off, of course."

"I know there'll be lots of family there on Tuesday, *comadre*. I'm not going in until after dinner time so you two can come home early and rest. What about Gil, do you want him to stay overnight with us?"

"I'll ask him, *comadre*. Manuel has offered to have him over because of little Manuel. Maybe I'll let him do that."

"Anyway, *comadre*," I assured her, "I'm planning to stay most of the night on Tuesday just in case the girls need anything. I always like to be in the room as much as possible when someone is in the hospital. You never know if they'll need a glass of water or can't reach the nurse's buzzer. It'll be a long day for you, and I know you'll be back there early on Wednesday. So don't worry if you don't see me there during the day. I'll be there at night."

That was my rationalization to her. In reality, I knew that I'd be so nervous Tuesday night that I wouldn't be able to sleep anyway, so I might as well do something useful. I knew that I'd feel much better if I could see for myself how the girls got through the night, whether they'd get fevers or suffer other complications. I wanted to be on the spot and not hear anything secondhand.

Maggie glanced my way. "*Comadre*, you don't have to do that, but whatever makes you feel comfortable is all right. I'll call you as soon as they're out of surgery and we have the doctor's report."

"Oh, good, *comadre*. Thank you."

Monday passed and Tuesday finally arrived. Normally, I don't like napping in the middle of the day because it makes me feel that I'll miss something. But on that Tuesday, I lay down about one-thirty in the afternoon to try and sleep, since I wasn't expecting to get much rest at night. Sleep never came. I looked at my watch at regular intervals, antsy at not being able to nod off. Finally, I told myself, "It doesn't matter. Just lying down and resting is important. Got to get some rest for tonight."

Shut eyelids sure don't guarantee sleep. My brain felt wide awake, and I kept repeating, "Don't think, don't think, don't think."

Eventually, I heard a key turn in the front door as one of the kids came home from school. The second one arrived shortly afterwards. They knew I was home because my car was in the driveway. I heard their footsteps on the stairs to the family room, back into the kitchen, then on the stairs leading to the bedrooms. Our bedroom door cracked open, then shut again.

I feigned sleep, still hoping it would come. Whispers followed the steps back downstairs. Their dad routinely went into work early and returned early—about three-thirty. I heard the garage door opener signal his arrival and the footfalls on the carpet as Joe and Cynthia hurried down to meet him. More whispering. Just as I'd decided napping was futile and tossed off the coverlet, Lupe and the kids opened the bedroom door.

"What's the matter, hon? Don't you feel well? Is everything okay?" he asked.

The kids were right behind him and squeezed past him in order to reach me. They looked worried.

"Yes, it's okay. I'm all right. I feel fine, *mijos*. It's just that I'm going up to the hospital tonight after dinner and I don't know how long I'll be there, so I wanted to take a little nap, that's all." I reached out to get my after school hugs.

Joe said, "Well, it's just that you never sleep during the day. We thought maybe you didn't feel good." Turning to his sister, he said, "See, I told you Mom was okay."

Relief spread across Cynthia's face, and I gave her an extra hug.

"Hey, you want a snack?" I asked.

Joe and Cynthia changed from their school uniforms into play clothes. After their snack they went out in front of the cul-de-sac to play with our neighbors' children. Playing with the other kids in the neighborhood was a much-awaited routine.

True to her word, Maggie called us from the hospital during dinner to say that all had gone well and both the girls were out of post-op and resting in their rooms. For kidney transplant surgery, the donor and the recipient need different levels of care and are kept in different rooms. Maggie sounded relieved, but sapped of her usual energy.

"*Gracias a Dios*," escaped from both of us.

I left for the hospital about six-thirty. Lupe stayed home with the kids and made sure that they finished their homework and took their showers. Knowing how important this was to me, the kids made no protest at my departure.

"I'll call you from the hospital after I find out what's going on," I told him.

"That's fine, honey. Be careful driving. Have one of the security people walk you out to the car. Call me before you leave, okay?"

It seemed like it took me longer to find a parking space in the congested lot than it did to drive up to the city. Finding my way around the maze of hospital corridors seemed even more time consuming. Impatiently I trekked along, feeling like a hiker exploring unknown territory, not knowing where the road ended. As I walked down what I hoped was the last hallway on the seventh floor, I encountered Maggie, Mando, Manuel, and his wife, Chavela, close cousins and camping mates, heading towards me. Everyone looked dragged out.

"*Comadre*," Maggie said as she opened up her arms.

I returned her embrace. "Everything still all right? How's Terri, Sylvia?"

Maggie nodded several times. "Yes, yes, it's fine. Terri's doing good and so is Sylvia. The kidney took, *comadre*, the kidney took." Joyful tears fell.

"*Gracias a Dios*" was the best I could do as I stifled my own tears.

Mando, too, looked exhausted but relieved. We all greeted each other and said goodbye at the same time. I went into Sylvia's room first. She was asleep. An IV with two bags fed into her arm. Other than that, she looked tranquil. When I kissed her forehead, it felt cool. I lifted one of the guest chairs over to her side and eased into it. The peaceful silence was calming and reassuring. She did look fine. The worried creases on her forehead were gone, and the rhythmic breathing was music to my ears.

I glanced about the room. A young man's picture was on her night-stand, and I wondered who it was. Mainly, I watched her breathing. She was so serene, almost as if her body, relieved of its distress, was renewing itself. My fears evaporated and I said a silent prayer of thanksgiving.

At the nurses' station, I asked for Terri's room number and was told to stay for only a few minutes. Terri's tousled curls made a lovely frame about her face. She was sound asleep, as her nurse had said she would be. We'd been told by the doctors that this type of surgery is harder on the donor than it is on the recipient. I almost dreaded entering her room for fear of what I'd find.

My apprehension dissolved when I noticed what seemed like normal, regular breathing. There was a slight frown on her brow, a puzzled look, as if she was having a bewildering dream. I wanted to hug and kiss her to pieces. With great restraint, I controlled myself and, assured that she was resting well, returned to Sylvia's room.

I alternated between sitting, standing and looking out the window through a space I'd opened up in the drapes. Since there was very little light in the room, some of the outside was visible but not scenic. Fans on top of the lower roof twirled monotonously. The fog was a fine mist tonight. Tall pines were visible from Golden Gate Park. All was hushed. No sirens or loud voices came from the streets. Visiting hours were over, and the hospital noises became muted as activity switched to the grave-yard shift. No one came to ask me to leave, so I remained, hoping Sylvia might wake up, at the same time hoping she wouldn't. I wanted to hear her voice, see her smile, but I knew that healing was enhanced by rest.

A nurse slipped in at one point, giving me a brief nod before check-ing the bags on the IV pole. I whispered, "How is she doing?"

"Are you a relative?" she asked.

"Oh yes, I'm her aunt and godmother. Her parents are my in-laws, and we're all really close."

She seemed satisfied. "Sylvia's doing very well. Her creatinine levels are getting better, no fever. She's making urine. So far, so good."

I wasn't quite sure what creatinine was, but if the levels were good, it made me happy. My breast filled with relief and thankfulness. It was like reaching an oasis after being lost in the desert. Sylvia had her life back, and the joy was indescribable.

About eleven o'clock, it was obvious I wasn't needed. Neither girl needed a cool towel for her forehead or a squeeze to the hand. The very capable, professional support watching over them was more than enough to instill confidence in anyone that their every need was being met. I left with a light and tranquil heart. It seemed our miracle was now solid fact.

A few days later, the mystery of the picture of the young man on Sylvia's hospital stand was solved. It turned out to be a picture of Terri's boyfriend, Chano, who lived out of town. Sylvia had taken it from Terri's room and instructed her mom to put it on her nightstand prior to sur-gery. After surgery, when Terri was in shape to visit Sylvia in her room, she was surprised to see Chano staring her in the face.

"What's he doing here?" she accused.

"Oh, Terri," Sylvia heaved dramatically. "Every time my kidney sees him, it sighs."

"*Cabrona*! Give it here." Terri snatched it off the stand while laughing at her sister's antics. "You must be all right if you can come up with this." Chano switched rooms.

The term "*cabrón*" or "*cabrona*" is used in our families as a term of endearment, much like saying "brat" or "stinker." In other families it can have a rude connotation and is considered to be insulting. We, however, use it freely with our children when they're being naughty, funny, silly, mischievous, or ill-behaved and we want them to stop such conduct. Under such circumstances, no offense is intended, as those words are not used in anger. It's never used in any other context except as an endearing reproach.

As far as Sylvia's prank was concerned, we loved it. Naturally, every time we had Terri and Sylvia in the same room, one of the *tíos* would ask Sylvia, "Say, *mija*. Is your kidney still sighing over Chano?"

We extracted a lot of mileage from Sylvia's joke. Most of all, it was so good to be laughing again.

Terri came home about eight days after the surgery, a bit sore and slow to move. Sylvia stayed in a couple of extra days to make sure her new kidney was functioning properly and to find the right dosages for the new medications she needed to take. All organ recipients need to take immunosuppressants to prevent the body's rejection of what it reacts to as a foreign object.

Once that concern was resolved, Sylvia came home, back on the road to resuming a normal life. As were the rest of us, especially Maggie and Mando, who were back to their old selves. Occasionally, Sylvia needed an adjustment to her meds. But gradually those times diminished and a familiar, welcome routine slipped into place.

Sylvia's face was back to its fine features, and the lightness in her step returned. She became animated again, and it was hard to believe how seriously ill she'd been such a short time ago. Terri bounced back with youthful exuberance, and four weeks after their surgery, an outsider would never have believed that these two young women had endured anything out of the ordinary. If I or anyone else tried to express appreciation to Terri and say how much her generous action meant to us, she still shrugged it off.

"Oh, *tia*. It wasn't anything. It was worth it, and look at me, I'm the same. Most of the time, I forget I've only got the one kidney." And out shot her famous cackle.

To look at her, she was right. On the outside, there wasn't any visible sign of anything missing, except for the long scar around her waist, which didn't show. Inside was another matter. It must have been akin to giving birth, for there was no doubt that she'd gifted her sister with an extended life. At least, that's how we looked at it. Terri became even more special to us.

Although she and Sylvia had always been close, a different level in their relationship became apparent. The kidding and teasing never stopped. But from that time forward, neither one ever seemed to get really upset with the other. I never heard Sylvia say anything derogatory about Terri or do anything that might not be completely supportive of her sister. When greater tragedy struck, that characteristic would become even stronger.

It appeared that we had a happy ending to our traumatic family crisis. Surely our portion of misfortune had been satisfied. As it turned out, it was simply a respite. A greater calamity awaited Maggie, her children and those of us who were part of them.

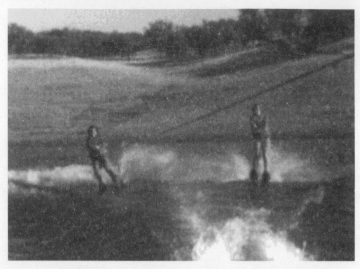

Summer of 1981 at Lake Don Pedro, CA.
Cynthia (left) and Sylvia skiing behind our boat.

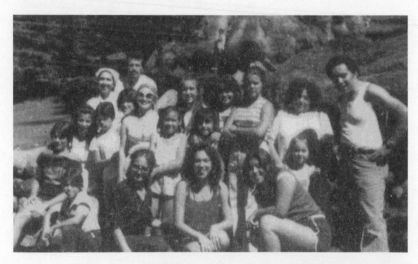

Labor Day Weekend 1981 visit to Yosemite National Park, CA, near
Lake Don Pedro. The Camping Gang: Joe Zertuche, Jr. is in second row
far left and Sylvia is directly behind him with her arm across his upper
chest. Cynthia is in the second row, third from the right. Bel is in second
row, fourth from left with sunglasses. The others are close family friends.

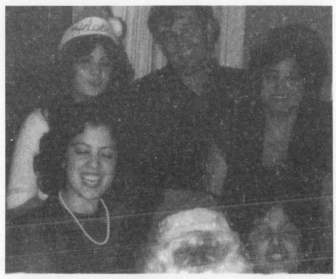

Armando and Maggie Zertuche's family with Santa: Gilbert, bottom right, Terri, bottom left, Sylvia wearing a "Santa's Helper" hat at upper left next to Mando and Maggie.

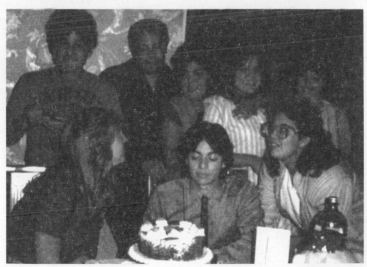

Joe's 19th Birthday, June 22, 1984, one day after Sylvia's birthday. Gathered in our dining room: Bottom left, Patty (Joe's Jr.'s friend) Joe, Jr. at center, Terri to Joe's right. Second row: from left: Gilbert, Joe, Sr., Sylvia with arm around Cynthia, Cynthia, and a friend. Note Sylvia's swollen face from the Prednisone.

59

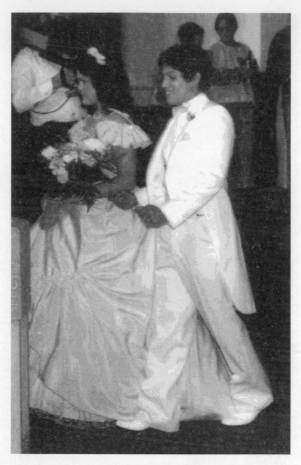

Cynthia's quinceañera, February 1984, St. Veronica's Church, South San Francisco. Cousin Gilbert Zertuche is her escort. They are about to place a bouquet of flowers at a Statue of Our Lady, a traditional homage.

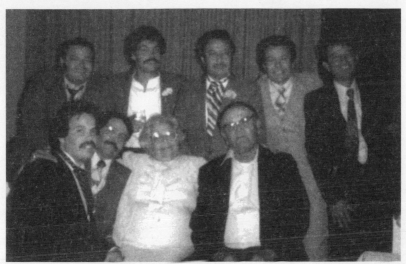

The Zertuche sons with their parents, Maria Zertuche and Matias Zertuche, seated in center. Taken in July 1984 at the wedding reception of nephew John Zertuche (Serjio's son) at the Morelos Hall in South San Francisco. Groom John is at bottom left, son Robert, Maria, Matias. Second Row: Sons Enrique, Carlos, Serjio, Joe, Sr. and Armando (Sylvia's dad).

7

Dreams Turn to Nightmares

A close group of four or five of our families continued to enjoy frequent jaunts to Turlock Lake campsite most summer weekends and for vacations. Several peripheral families, friends and relatives joined us from time to time, increasing the youth population to over a dozen. Camping, boating and water skiing were the recreational activities of choice, and it was a great time for the kids as well as the adults.

We watched the Lake Don Pedro area start to develop as realty companies began selling acreage lots for vacation homes. A half-block commercial area sprung up boasting a rustic, western architectural façade. The hills around the lake sprouted a few summer homes. Freshly asphalted streets zigzagged through the golden hills surrounding the lake in readiness for the anticipated population growth.

Lupe and I started to scout around for a parcel that might be suitable for a retirement place. We eventually found two adjoining parcels that had a marvelous view of the lake. Abutting the Turlock Irrigation District's green belt at the shoreline, the lots had unhampered views and access to the water. Our plan was to hold them until retirement age approached, then we'd start working on building plans. At the time of our purchase in 1982, we were about twenty-five years from that objective.

Just as Lupe and I thought we had our lives on course, Lupe's employer, Dupont Company, announced that they were closing down their South City plant in 1983. He had started working for Dupont in 1966, nine months after Joe was born. At forty-seven, Lupe was too young to retire, and the thought of looking for a new job was demoralizing to him. We considered moving to one of the out-of-state Dupont plants (as they offered), but Joe was a junior in high school. If we moved, I would have stayed behind for one year until he graduated with his class. Neither his dad nor I wanted to live separately for a year, so we decided not to move out of California.

I remember the desperate look in Lupe's eyes as he scanned the want ads in the newspapers, and I remember my attempts to encourage him.

"Don't worry, hon. I know you'll find something. We have a little in the bank. I've got my part-time job. You'll get some severance pay. We'll be all right."

He looked up from the kitchen table, set down the paper to light up a cigarette and nodded. He was humoring me without believing me. I knew that the uncertainty of our financial security weighed heavily on him. While I was concerned, I had a lot of faith in my husband, in his skills, and was confident that eventually he'd land a good job.

However, after a few weeks of earnest looking without results, his apprehension began to rub off on me. Now I was looking in the paper for jobs he might be interested in. One day my boss, a wealthy business entrepreneur from a California pioneer family, asked, "Bel, I heard that Dupont was closing. Isn't that where your husband works?"

I never discussed personal family affairs outside our home or family. Yet the tone in Mr. McAllister's voice was filled with genuine concern, so I opened up a bit.

"Yes, Mr. McAllister, it is."

"So, what's happening?"

"Well, the company has offered transfers to their out-of-state locations. But he's looking for a job in this area."

He straightened up in his chair, looking very healthy and distinctive for a seventy-eight-year-old. "You're not going to move, are you? Oh, don't do that. Let me ask around." He courteously added, "If you don't mind, that is."

Mind? I could have jumped up and hugged him. Instead I said, "That would be wonderful, sir. We'd appreciate it."

No more time was wasted on small talk. He was a real dynamo, and every minute was dedicated to working at full speed so that he could leave the office at noon for his club on Nob Hill. That evening, I didn't mention Mr. McAllister's comment to Lupe because I didn't want to get his hopes up. I hardly dared to hope myself.

The following week, Mr. McAllister had a job offer for Lupe at Varian & Associates in Palo Alto. He sat on their board. When he told me, I couldn't believe it. I barely managed a choked thank you before he slid a note across the desk. "Here's the man he has to call for an interview. It's in the furnace division. Shouldn't be a problem with your husband's background at Dupont. Now, what needs following up today?"

As it turned out, while Lupe was grateful to be employed, he hated the job. Dupont was ten minutes from our house. Varian & Associates was forty-five minutes in heavy traffic. He also missed his Dupont buddies. Adding insult to injury, he earned less. He counted the days until he could retire.

In those days, a first cousin of mine, Manny, visited us often. We'd always been real tight. He'd also been looking for a job for a few months, and it wasn't unusual for him and Lupe to commiserate over coffee and cigarettes after dinner. Frustrated at not finding a new job, Manny said he'd made a decision. "I'm thinking of looking for a little business I can buy."

Without skipping a beat, Lupe countered, "Yeah, that's the thing to do. Say, you've got the time to look. You look. Let me know if you find anything, and maybe we can go in together."

I was at the kitchen counter preparing school lunches for the kids. "Like what, cuz?"

"I don't know. Maybe a hardware store. Hey, Lupe, you're pretty handy. What about a chain of laundry stores? Yeah, you don't have to be there much, and if anything goes wrong with the machines, you can fix 'em. Between the two of us, we can get several of 'em."

"I could do that," Lupe said enthusiastically.

After Manny left, I asked, "Are you serious about this business thing, hon? You know you'll have to be able to work with Manny. You think you can do that?"

"I think so. I think we could make it. I know how he is, and I'd keep on top of things. I sure would like to get out of that place."

I dropped the subject, thinking nothing would ever come of it. I couldn't have been more mistaken.

On Labor Day weekend Manny drove up to Lake Don Pedro. We found him waiting for us at the campground when we returned from water skiing. He never came up, so we were really surprised to see him. I hoped nothing was wrong. Not yet, there wasn't.

Manny drew us aside and was really excited. "You won't believe this, cuz. I bumped into Juan Diaz downtown last week. We got to talkin', and he tells me that he's selling the Silver Dollar. So, Friday and Saturday nights I go down there. He's got this great salsa band, ten guys, really great, wear tuxes, and do they pack 'em in. I'm tellin' ya, it's standing room only! It's a gold mine!"

Lupe's ears pointed straight up.

"A nightclub? Are you nuts, Manny?" I said. "You know how much work that is? Besides, he probably wants a fortune for the place."

We all knew Juan Diaz and the Silver Dollar, a place in downtown South City that we avoided because it didn't have a good reputation. But Lupe asked me if we could check it out the following weekend. I agreed because Lupe was so good about supporting me whenever I suggested a financial move. I figured it was my turn to do the same. That weekend Manny, Lupe and I went down to Diaz' place. One look at the burgeoning Saturday night throng waiting to get in turned Lupe's pupils into dollar signs. Juan Diaz spotted us, comped the cover charge and bought us drinks. By the time we left, he, Manny and Lupe had agreed to have coffee on Sunday afternoon. I declined the invitation, preferring to be with the kids.

"Don't worry, hon," Lupe said. "I just want to see what he has to offer. We don't even know what he's asking for it. Hey, did you notice that the building has rooms upstairs? That has to bring in some good rent."

"A nightclub?" I shrugged. "I can't imagine us in a nightclub."

"Well, we're not there yet. Manny's pretty revved up about it, though. I'll just go along with him to hear for myself what Juan has to say."

I relied on Lupe's assurance that he was just exploring the possibilities of the venture and thought we were on the same wavelength. Not so. We signed escrow papers December 12th, the feast day of La Virgen de Guadalupe. Nine months later, Lupe and I were separated; thirteen months later we were in divorce proceedings. His mantra had become, "Nothing and no one is more important to me than the business. I *have* to be there!" And he followed it to the fullest. I never knew what happened to the man I'd married. Some stranger now occupied his body, and the heartbreak of my old Lupe's absence was excruciating.

At the time I was so emotionally crushed that it was all I could do to place one foot in front of the other to carry on. It was bad enough losing Lupe to the business, but having my family broken up was against everything I'd ever wanted out of life. It would take years before the realization that my family had not been broken up sunk in. Joe, Cynthia and I remained a loving, strong, functioning unit. Nothing would ever rob us of that. But in those early days of my separation from their dad, I relied heavily on the only Father I've ever known for comfort. I accepted the cross that God had sent, but pleaded for the strength to bear it. As usual, He did provide it, although at the time, it didn't seem enough.

Anyone who's gone through divorce knows how painful it is. I tried to be strong for Joe and Cynthia, she being more deeply affected by her father's leaving than her brother. My job went from part-time to full-time. While the Zertuche clan rallied beside me and insisted on keeping me in the fold, I still felt stripped of my former family life. It was a horrific loss. With the help of supportive family and friends (especially my pals, Kate and Kitty), I survived to forge a new life. Unfortunately, my *comadre*'s nightmare was still to come.

While I was going through my divorce, the rest of the Zertuches carried on with their normal routines. One of the cousins, Manuel Bernal, purchased a lot outside of the town of Atwater, in close proximity to Lake Don Pedro. He started erecting a vacation home. Mando and other family members gave him a hand in their free time. Later, Manuel and our *compadres* acquired a large parcel of land, about 20 acres, closer to the lake. Theirs was a partnership formed first from family ties; secondly, from a genuine friendship that had grown stronger during the last decade. Before long, the two couples were talking about developing their property, each occupying half of the acreage.

Aside from the goal of building their dream house, Mando and Maggie explored the possibility of starting a chicken farm and sought professional business advice about it. They also talked about adding pigs and a few goats to the mix, enough to generate an income that would permit Mando to retire early. They were convinced that they could not only sustain themselves, but also make their *ranchito* a profitable venture. Naturally, they were very excited about the prospects. Maggie had always expressed a love for country living.

"*Un ranchito*," as she wishfully referred to it.

And Mando was one hundred per cent in agreement. Plans accelerated, and before the rest of us fully digested the impending move, they'd placed their South City home on the market. In retrospect, I think that the thought of their moving from the tight circle in which we lived seemed unbelievable, or we wished it to be unbelievable. Once the probability became fact, we were happy for them because they were so happy for themselves.

When their home sold, they purchased a comfortable mobile home from which they could watch their plans take form. Perched atop a golden hillcrest on their own ten-acre portion, they observed the beginning of this grand dream. The necessary building permits were obtained, the pad was excavated, and installation of the power poles awaited. Mando was able to change jobs in order to be closer to the new home site. Plans for his early retirement seemed enticingly possible as construction activity began in earnest. At the time it seemed like their future held nothing but promise. It was a dreadful deception.

Anyone who's ever built a house or even added on to an existing one knows how frustrating the requirements for permits and building requisites can be. In this case, the utility company was being a major thorn in Mando's side. As was later explained to me, one Monday evening in mid-November, he arrived at the mobile home expecting to find that the utility company had hooked up power to the lines for the new house.

"Well, did they show up?" he asked.

At the stove finishing dinner, Maggie shook her head and spoke while her hands continued with the all-too-familiar motions that went into feeding her family. "Well, they did come, but they said that they didn't have the right paperwork or someone didn't sign off right, so they couldn't go ahead…" Maggie's voice, edged with frustration, was interrupted before she could finish.

Mando shouted, "What!" Several expletives bounced off the walls of the compact kitchen. "They were supposed to do that today, without fail! That holds up everything!" He ranted and vented. He was fuming, not at any person in particular, but at the frustrating situation. It seemed he was constantly bucking either the County Building Division or the utility company. You'd think he was asking for a permit to build a nuclear power plant, he claimed. His gut roiled as he anticipated another discussion with whoever was responsible for the latest glitch.

Dinner was unusually quiet. After he'd eaten, he was a bit calmer. He grabbed the newspaper and went into the living room to watch his favorite team, the San Francisco Forty-Niners, on Monday Night Football. Shortly after he'd sat down, a wave of pain shot through him and a yell pierced the mobile home. Maggie, Gil and the girls rushed out of the kitchen. When Gil arrived at his father's side, he immediately applied CPR. Someone called the emergency number. Despite Gil's efforts and those of the emergency medical team, Mando died of what was thought to be a massive coronary at the age of forty-five that November in 1985.

Fate seems to take perverse pleasure in dogging the same family with repeated misfortune. This profound loss leveled Maggie and the children. Its impact was shattering.

Despite the divorce, Lupe and I maintained a civil channel of communication, especially in matters pertaining to the children or family. Though I tried to limit our conversations, it wasn't unusual for me to call him at the Silver Dollar. On the evening when my mother-in-law called with the terrible news, she asked that I call Lupe to let him know about his brother since she had more calls to make. I agreed.

"What! Mando! Are you sure?" I could hear the jukebox playing in the background mingled with the rowdy voices of patrons. I could picture the scene and almost smell the smoke hazing the dimly lit bar area. The large dance floor in the back would be empty since it only saw activity on weekends. In my mind I could see the chairs piled on top of the tiny cocktail tables, waiting for the next onslaught of drinking dancers. During the week, a few of the regulars would be seated at the long front bar or playing darts. I'd hated the nine months I worked there. Even over the telephone, the mere sound of the ambiance churned my stomach. Lupe, on the other hand, thrived in that atmosphere.

I assured him that the news was true and relayed what details there were to share about Mando's death, including the fact that Manuel and Charlie, Lupe's youngest brother, were on their way up to get Maggie and the kids.

I could tell how shocked he was. "I'll go up, too. What time is it? Eight o'clock. I'll have Beto close up. What time is Charlie leaving? Maybe I can catch a ride with him."

I offered to call my cousin Maria, Charlie's wife, to see if he had left yet. It turned out he'd already left. I called Lupe back to tell him. I'm not sure if he ever left the bar to go to the lake; all I knew was that Maggie and the kids were on their way to Serjio's, as was I.

It was about a three-hour drive from South City to the lake, and my *compadres'* place was just beyond that by a few more miles. The round trip took over six hours. Manuel brought Maggie to Serjio's house, and Terri followed, driving Sylvia and Gil down. The mood inside the car must have been somber. By the time I arrived at Serjio's, Sylvia, Terri and Gilbert had left to go to their grandparents' house, although both Maria and Matias were at Serjio's trying to comfort the new widow.

Entering Serjio and Josie's house, I went to the back family room where everyone was gathered. My in-laws, my mother-in-law's older brother, Hilario, and a couple of close friends sat around the game table or in easy chairs. Maggie lay slumped on the couch, her head tilted all the way back. I can't recall seeing a more desolate human being. Repetitive sobs of, "Ayy, ayy, *Viejo, Viejo*." pierced my ears, cutting me to the quick. "*Viejo*" means "my old man" in Spanish and is more of an endearing term than it may sound, similar to the hippie days when young couples referred to each other as "my old lady" or "my old man." Mando had lovingly called her his *Vieja*.

Her heart was ripped apart. Her voice carried her anguish. I slipped onto the couch next to her, but she didn't see or hear me as I offered useless words. Her hands were ice cold, and her head rolled from side to side on the top edge of the sofa, eyes shut, sobbing, moaning, repeating his name. A handkerchief pressed against her mouth muffled some of her grief.

"Why did you leave me? *Dios mio, por que, por que?*" Unabated sorrow poured out. She went on for hours. We tried to get her to drink a shot of whiskey, a cup of coffee, tea, anything, to no avail.

No one in the room had more information on Mando's death other than it had been sudden and so final. Someone repeated that Gil had immediately tried mouth-to-mouth resuscitation on his father, but by the time the paramedics arrived, Mando was gone.

The scene was surreal. Maria, Hilario, Matias and I sat at the table with cold cups of coffee in front of us. Maria had lost her son, yet her own grief seemed placed on hold. No tears stained her face, and she was amazingly calm. I wondered at this degree of calm, not knowing whether to admire it or question it. On one hand, it struck me as too unnatural. On the other hand, it might have been an attempt to stabilize emotions within the room. Whatever the cause, I concluded that it was best not to be judgmental in instances like these. I watched as she lit up a menthol Salem cigarette. Her eyes followed the rising, curling smoke. What is she feeling, thinking? I wondered.

Primal fear was in the room. Perhaps because we realized that fate hadn't stricken us. Serjio and Josie were robotic hosts, going through the correct movements. Serjio and Mando were probably the closest of the six brothers, and Mando's death had created an emptiness at his side, like a missing limb.

Matias occasionally bowed his head to cover his face with his hands. Was he crying? I couldn't tell, but I could sense his feeling of loss. Collectively, we shuddered at the impact this tragedy held for Maggie and her family. My Sylvia adored her father. Terri, his first-born, idolized him. Gil's efforts to win his dad's approval played in my mind, and I hoped that Gil knew how much his dad had really loved him.

No matter how much I tried to suppress the thought, I was frightened at the emotional and financial toll Mando's death would have on my *comadre*. They had no home—either in South City or at the lake. What a horrendous tragedy. At the moment, we could only turn to the practical matters of assisting with funeral arrangements.

Our custom was to have two nights at the funeral home's chapel. The first night was usually just a wake; the second night included the saying of the rosary and a homily by a priest. The mortuary was packed with all of South City's Mexican community as well as our American friends and city officials. All were grieved and shocked at the unexpected loss of someone in the prime of life. Mando was put to rest at Holy Cross Cemetery after a requiem Mass. Many relatives and even more friends came out to memorialize the young husband, father, son, brother and friend. Maggie was overwhelmed with condolences and offers of help. Sadly, what she needed was not within our power to give.

During the first days following Mando's death, Maggie, Terri, Sylvia and Gilbert bravely endured all the people around them. Kind words, sympathy and condolences poured in. The parade of relatives and friends prevented me from getting close enough to sit with Sylvia on a one-on-one basis, and I sensed the timing was wrong. She was too distraught to push it. Both she and Terri were quiet, making the right responses, nodding to acknowledge condolences, speaking softly because their heartache used up so much space. I observed them whispering and knew how often they sought the solitary consolation of their bedroom in Grandma Maria's house. Although I attempted to comfort all three children as best I could, it was such an emotionally raw time that nothing seemed enough or adequate.

Eventually, relatives from Southern California and the many friends who had come to pay their respects started to disband and return to their daily lives. There was no normalcy for Maggie and her family. Four lives were immersed in grief, shock and confusion. Financial uncertainty made every day a nightmare. My *comadre's* grief hardened into stoicism.

"Why, *nina*? Why my daddy?" Sylvia sobbed. "What did he ever do to deserve to die?" I had no answers for her.

Terri worried me more because I didn't see her cry. If she did, I didn't see it. It worried me that she was withdrawing. Actions and conversations indicated that Maggie had become Terri's cause. Both she and Sylvia watched over and comforted their mother as best they could. I observed a pattern of protective conduct between them and witnessed its gradual evolution into an unspoken pact of responsibility that enveloped their mother. Perhaps it was a solemn promise to the memory of their father and, in his stead, they now assumed the role of care he'd been so good at. They were about to take over as joint heads of the family, and Maggie would continue as its heart. But it wasn't easy when they, too, were in need of comfort.

There was no other recourse but for Maggie and the kids to move in with the in-laws. Fortunately, the house was big enough, and with only two sons living at home, Maggie, Terri and Sylvia had their own bedrooms. Gil shared a room with one of his younger uncles, and for a few weeks, the transition seemed to work. However, there's an old saying in Spanish that says guests and fish begin to smell after three days. Unfortunately, Maggie began to experience the truth of that saying in her mother-in-law's house all too soon. Tolerance of her and her children shortly fell into what appeared to be the category of unwanted guests for Maria.

Matias, on the other hand, loved having them in his home. Of all the daughters-in-law, Maggie got along the best with our father-in-law. She knew just how to talk to him and cleverly dodged his unpolished manners and speech with sassy retorts that tickled him. Without lack of respect, she could carry a on conversation with him, *mano a mano*, and end it still friends. I've always thought that this kinship Maggie shared with our *suegro* struck pangs of jealousy within Maria. Add the ingredient of two women in the same kitchen, and you have a situation like this one.

There seemed no doubt that Maria resented having to share her husband and domain with her husband's favorite daughter-in-law. And as the weeks passed, Maggie, Terri, Sylvia and Gil were becoming silently uncomfortable.

Even after the divorce, I was still very welcome at the Zertuche house. And my ex-*suegra* often called me to stop by after work or on the weekend for a visit. This habit of hers remained true until her death. On Sundays after Mass, I'd usually stop by for a few moments to drop Cynthia off so that she could spend some time with Terri, Sylvia and Gil. If her dad was at the house, I'd save my visit for another time. Not because of any acrimony, I just felt that he was entitled to feel comfortable in his parents' home. When Terri and Sylvia were there we had a good visit before they took the "brat" out on their forays to fast-food restaurants, the movies or visiting friends. The atmosphere appeared courteous, but when Maggie and the girls weren't present, my mother-in-law shared petty complaints with me.

Rattling in Spanish, she vented. "I can't find any of my sewing patterns with Maggie straightening up all the time. Hmphff, she cleans and displaces all my things. Always cleaning, constantly rearranging. I can't find anything! I used to be able to put my finger on anything I wanted. Now I have to hunt for it." Her outrage sounded harsher in Spanish. Maria puffed at her cigarette.

"*Suegra*, she's just trying to be helpful." To myself I thought that the house had never looked so nice.

"And Maria Teresa! She gets anything she wants." Another heavy drag on her ever-present cigarette. "She has your *suegro* wrapped around her little finger." Mimicking Terri's voice, she said, "Grandpa, I want this, I want that." With indignation, she added, "And he gets it for her!"

Aha, I thought. There lies the problem. Her territory is being in-fringed upon. It was hard to sympathize with the lack of understanding that this old woman possessed. Wasn't gray hair accompanied by wis-dom? Who should have had greater compassion for a widow than the mother of the deceased son? It was an incomprehensible situation to me. And in the back of my mind, it's always bothered me that I never saw her shed a tear for Mando.

At Maggie's request, cousin Manuel had sold the twenty-acre parcel at the lake and divided the proceeds according to the partnership they had had when Mando was alive. Fortunately, due to Manuel's efforts, it sold quickly considering that vacant land doesn't sell as fast as actual houses. By this time, Maggie's uneasiness with living with her mother-in-law was obvious and becoming more difficult.

Maggie would come over to my house for coffee, sometimes with Terri and Sylvia, other times without. At first, we went over Mando's insurance papers and the like to make sure that all assets had surfaced. We made an appointment to go to the Social Security office in Daly City, only to be told that the $250 death benefit was all that the widow was entitled to and that Mando's Social Security benefits would not be re-ceived until she was at least sixty-two. Because Gil was under eighteen, she'd receive a small allotment for him. It would promptly disappear when he turned eighteen in less than two years.

If I was surprised by the cold facts meted out by the Social Security office, Maggie was really taken aback. Every time she turned around, it seemed she was confronted with bad news. I couldn't believe the clerk when she delivered this latest blow. When we walked out of the office, we were both disheartened. I wondered how much more could she take.

8

Relocating Without Mando

The city of Stockton is part of California's Central Valley, an agricultural Mecca and, during the exciting gold rush days, an important, bustling port. At present the port is less busy, but in the seventies and eighties residential developers discovered the lure of Stockton's land for home construction. House-starved Bay Area residents fueled the building boom. In comparison to the immediate San Francisco Bay Area, life is less expensive, especially the cost of homes, which have rapidly supplanted orchards, lettuce fields, corn and cattle-grazing territory. Their affordable prices attract hordes from all over Northern California. A $200,000 house there would cost two or three times as much in the San Francisco Bay Area, which meant that Stockton in 1985 was the new land of milk and honey if you wanted to buy an affordable house.

Santa Clara County's Silicon Valley was booming. As plants and office buildings displaced prune yards, orchards and farmlands in their own county, the workforce hungered to buy their own homes. Rural areas like Stockton, Lodi and Modesto quickly became bedroom communities with great economic appeal. Commuting the long distances from the Stockton-Modesto area to the San Jose area was the necessary price for the privilege of paying property taxes, as congested traffic headaches substantiated.

It turned out that Maggie's younger brother and his family had moved to Stockton within the two years prior to Mando's death. From the early days of her young widowhood, he encouraged Maggie to move there. "You'll be closer to your own family, *hermana* (sister). At least, come up and take a look."

With the unsatisfactory situation at the in-laws', it was inevitable that such an escape route would tempt Maggie and the girls. They looked at some new housing developments in Stockton and pondered the possibilities of such a move. Naturally, it'd be a big change, but preferable to the current situation. So, with the proceeds derived from the sale of the Don Pedro Lake acreage, Maggie purchased an almost-new, three-bedroom, two-bath rancher with a family room and generous yard.

It was a bittersweet challenge for the new widow. The courage to buy and move into their first house without Mando must have called on Herculean resolve and super emotional strength. While it was liberating to escape from the in-laws' house, it was an additional, painful reminder that a new life without her *viejo* was beginning, and the awful fact of his absence struck anew. This harsh reality appeared to prompt the four to huddle even closer together, bunkering defensively against the world that was so hard on them. It was a tremendous decision and I'm sure very difficult. With great courage and amid the hustle of gathering their belongings, packing and moving, they shaped a new direction in life.

Sylvia and Terri matured beyond their years within those few months after their father's death. Gilbert seemed to be struggling more with all the changes. A steely determination developed that together they would face the world and shield their mother from as much as they could. It was as if Maggie had become their charge and they her protectors. It would have been beautiful to behold were it not for the heartache.

By doing what they felt needed to be done, Terri and Sylvia somehow conquered their collective fears and insecurity as well as the loneliness that must have lain just beneath the surface of their daily lives. Whether they relied on prayer or not, I don't know. Had their faith been shaken with Mando's death? It was too private a matter to bring up. I just made sure that they were in my daily prayers. Three women—one recently widowed, two fatherless—charged foreward to meet whatever lay ahead in a new town, with a new life in strange surroundings. As they settled, they turned the new house into a home, Terri and Sylvia found good jobs, and they settled into their new lives.

Both girls were employed in Stockton, and Maggie earned extra money by babysitting in her home. Life took on a different type of existence for them. While it was as good a life as could be managed, the adjustment must have fostered pangs for the days when Mando was in their midst. I imagine that sometimes that realization overshadowed the best of days. But overall, they found their footing and settled in place. From where I stood, it was quite an accomplishment, and I was so proud of them.

Gilbert hadn't followed his family to Stockton right away because he was still in school, and Maggie had decided that it was important for him to finish at his same high school in South City and graduate with his class. As a result, he stayed with me for a few months. It was nice having him around. He was never any trouble, emptied the garbage without being asked, picked up after himself and blended right in with us. Because they'd practically grown up together, he and my two got along famously. Our home was his, and I think he truly felt comfortable there.

Rightly or wrongly, he and I never talked about his dad's death. I hesitated to do so without Gil's initiating the topic. If he'd given me an opening, I'd have jumped in to give him an opportunity to release whatever emotions needed venting. But it seemed he wasn't ready or willing to share those feelings, and I respected that position. I often wondered if he and Joe or Cynthia ever discussed it. If they did, I was never aware of it.

When he first came to live with us, Terri did have one warning about her brother. "*Tia*, he takes really long showers." And she was right. Other than that, it was simply like having another son, one who really felt and acted like one. When his graduation day arrived, Maggie and the girls came down to see him get his diploma. Because of the limited tickets available, only they went. But we all gathered afterwards to celebrate while he went to his Grad Night at the high school gym. Terri and Sylvia stayed at our house, and it was great to see the girls interact and hear their banter again.

There was a lot going on at that time, because Cynthia was also a senior in high school and activities for her graduation were taking place. Mercy High School of Burlingame was holding the commencement ceremonies in San Francisco, and her dad, Joe and I were there to proudly witness the much-awaited handing out of the diplomas. I remembered how much my own graduation had meant to me, how I had thought it was the end of a tedious process and the beginning of a new type of freedom. I imagined seeing that same glimmering thought on Cynthia's face on her grad night.

I guess we all assumed that Gil would leave for Stockton as soon as the graduation parties were over, but he seemed reluctant to go. One day, I tried to find out why without laying a guilt trip on him.

"So, *mijo*, what do you think you'll be doing next?" I leaned back into the sofa cushions with my mug of coffee.

He and I were alone in the family room. How much had the trauma of seeing his dad die in front of him affected him, and in what and how many ways? There had to be lots there for him to deal with. I wanted to reach out, but wasn't quite sure how. Sitting on the edge of the couch, he stared down at the carpet, looking not at the pattern but somewhere beneath the fibers to a secret place that might have some answers.

"Gil, how are you feeling? Do you want to talk about anything? Do you want to stay here, go to Stockton? What's on your mind?"

I'd supposed that he was anxious to join his mother and sisters in Stockton. I guess we all figured that keeping the family in a cohesive unit was the natural thing to do. It plucked at my heartstrings to look at his pensive young face. Mando would have been so proud to see his son graduate. It was mid-morning, and his golden-brown hair was uncombed and a tousled mass of curls. His brown eyes flecked with gold seemed drained, empty. Indecisiveness marred his features.

"I don't know what I want to do, *tia*. I just don't know."

"Well, you're welcome to stay, Gil, you know that. Does moving up to Stockton make you a bit nervous?" I paused for some acknowledgement. When none came, I continued.

"That's understandable. I'm sure Terri and Sylvia were nervous about it, too. But you might want to give it a try. You could go to school up there, work part-time. You might find that you like it there. Your mom and the girls come down pretty often, and that would give you a chance to see the cousins and other friends. For that matter, they can go up there to see you since they're studying to get their driver's licenses. Hey, you'll be getting yours pretty soon, too."

My arm was about his shoulders and I gave him a squeeze. The weight of silence prevailed.

"Don't you think your mom and sisters would welcome your presence? It might be helpful. It could mean a lot to them, especially your mom. Have you talked about it with them?"

He still didn't look up, and I knew he wasn't going to open up those deep thoughts and feelings inside him. They were in his private safe deposit box, and he wasn't unlocking it. I didn't know how else to draw him out without making matters worse. So I said, "Well, give it some thought, *mijo*. You have a couple of options. Think about them. If you want to talk and toss them around, let me know. You might want to call Terri and get her take on it. Anytime you want to talk about it, let me know, *mijo*. I'll keep it to myself, you know that."

His response was a nod. The problem with not getting any feedback from your children is that you think the worst. My impression was that he felt overwhelmed by a need to be responsible, perhaps to take his father's place. In reality, Terri and Sylvia were carrying the major portion of the financial responsibility, and no one expected him to take over for his father.

Was he angry about his predicament? Who could blame him? Did he feel cheated by fate? Absolutely justified. Were some unknown plans quashed by his father's death? Whatever his feelings were, he kept them to himself, and I simply didn't have the expertise to draw them out, though I gave them much thought. It turned out that within a couple of weeks he did go up to Stockton, but it was to be a temporary arrangement.

Despite the distance, Sylvia and I retained our closeness. No one could say anything even slightly critical of me in front of her because she'd immediately jump all over them. "Don't you say anything about my *nina*. She's perfect."

Terri's imitation of her sister when she made that comment was hilarious and right on the mark. As a result of Sylvia's protectiveness toward me, she was constantly baited just to get her response.

During this time, Sylvia's transplanted kidney was functioning properly, and except for the need to take immunosuppressants and have routine check-ups, she was doing fine. She loved her job as administrative assistant at the Girl Scouts of America in Stockton, especially the people. She enjoyed talking to me about it. When alone, we shared our opinions. She vented about her siblings regarding minor things or talked about her dog, Freeway.

As the name implied, Mando had found him by the side of the freeway without dog tags and no one to claim him. So he brought him home. Freeway quickly became Sylvia's pet, friend and confidante, adding much joy to her life. I was thrilled that she had a replacement for Smokey, whose memory still touched me with guilt.

Sylvia and I thought so much alike. Our world was black and white, logical and funny. Most of all, funny. Her favorite reply, "Ay, *nina*," was music to my ears whenever we talked and exchanged opinions because it was uttered with an approving giggle.

Terri worked in a medical clinic where they made good use of her bilingual skills. She, Sylvia and my *comadre* became a tight unit, each pulling her own weight in building their new life. When old family friends had parties in South City, the girls would sometimes drive down. They still had great fun with their cousins and friends and were included in all that went on. Sometimes they didn't make the drive down. But when they did, it was great fun.

In 1989, Joe moved out of the house to move in with his cousin and another friend who'd rented a house in San Mateo. After all, he was twenty-four and it was time for him to leave the nest. Suddenly, the house seemed too big for just Cynthia and me. Additionally, with Joe gone, I did the yard work and general upkeep, which, together with holding down a full-time job, was more than I wanted to handle. Cynthia always helped with the housework, but I began to tire of having to spend half of my Saturday in the yard.

Stubbornness also played a part, I guess. I could have afforded a housekeeper twice a month, but I felt that it was important to set an example for Cynthia on the importance of keeping a clean house. In the process, I was wearing myself out and decided I had to find some resolution to all this weekend work. My housekeeping tactic was so effective that today my daughter employs a housekeeper! So much for setting good examples.

I started looking for a smaller house and was thrilled when I found a townhouse perched atop a hill in the adjacent town, San Bruno. The location was perfect and only fifteen minutes from my Burlingame office and close to our friends and families. All the outside work was done by the homeowners' association, and Cynthia and I each had our own master bedroom on different levels of the tri-level dwelling. It had a nice living area so that I could still host the family Thanksgiving dinner for my side of the family, which was my special holiday. And the view was awesome! The southern portion of the San Francisco Bay is visible from the living room windows, and a balcony next to the dining area provides views of Mount Diablo (weather permitting) and the East Bay. On a clear day you can see the San Mateo Bridge and across to Fremont. The airport sprawls to our left, and directly across the rear balcony is a protected watershed and open space area that greens the canyon and our vista.

The downside was that Cynthia had a very difficult time leaving the family home. It was an emotional upheaval for her. Once family and friends started coming over, including Sylvia and Terri, the strangeness of living in the townhouse versus her old home became more tolerable, although our old house still remains close to her heart. Luckily, I took out some of the equity from the family house and rented it out instead of selling it. Cynthia now lives there, next to the park where her precious Bailey (a mutt with beagle looks and tendencies) can run around.

One summer in the early nineties, Sylvia, Cynthia, and their younger cousin, Monica, took a vacation drive to Southern California. Matias' brother and sister-in-law, Chuey and Bertha, lived in Altadena, and the route from South City and Altadena had been traveled a lot through the years. When the kids were small and we drove our in-laws down for a visit or a wedding or other family function, *Tia* Bertha and *Tio* Chuey opened up their home to all of us. Wall-to-wall kids slept in the living room while the adults were given the bedrooms. Chuey rose every morning at five and made a huge batch of *tortillas de harina* (flour) for us. Bertha and her five daughters, mostly Terri and Sylvia's age, scrambled to help fix meals and play with the children. Laughter filled every nook of that house, and their hospitality was generous beyond belief.

The *tios* also came up to visit Matias and Maria on occasion, and many visitors to the in-laws' came to pay their respects whenever they were in town. Tio Chuey was as quiet and gentle as Matias was loud and gruff. With such opposite personalities, it was hard to believe that they were brothers.

Since the *tios* had hosted us so often in Southern California, all our children knew they could plan to stay with them and be received with open arms. So it was natural that Sylvia, Cynthia and Monica stayed with them on this particular trip. They used their *tios'* house as a base for a jaunt to Disneyland, a day-long shopping run into Tijuana, and other local trips. At night, when all the cousins (Chela, Hortencia, Juana Maria, Trini and Maggita) met for dinner at the house, the laughter was exceeded only by the quantity of food on the table. Cynthia took lots of photos on that trip attesting to the good times shared.

Sylvia was doing all the normal things that a twenty-nine-year-old does—working, playing and contributing to her household. On occasion, her medications needed adjustment, which was not unusual for a transplant recipient. Once they were fine-tuned, all was well again. Her creatinine levels were monitored on a regular basis, and she scheduled normal appointments with her doctors to make sure all aspects of her health were going smoothly.

A GIFT NOT WASTED

For ten years after her transplant surgery, her health routine flowed smoothly. She was generally well, working and playing. We were in the eleventh year of her transplant. At the time, we didn't suspect that Terri's donated kidney was nearing the end of its life span.

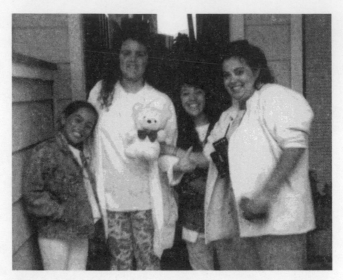

Cousins Rebeca and Erica Zertuche (Carlos Zertuche's daughters) in front of our townhouse with Cynthia and Sylvia, who took them to a New Kids on the Block concert in September 1990.

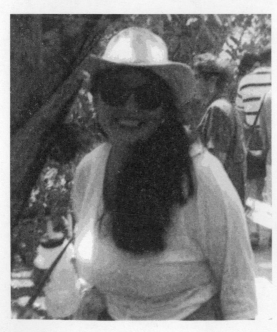

July 4, 1992, at Marine World Park, Vallejo, CA. Sylvia in white hat —she loved hats.

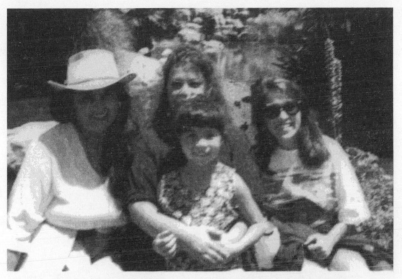

July 4, 1992, at Marine World Park, Vallejo, CA. Sylvia, Terri and cousin Erica. Little girl is a family friend, name unknown.

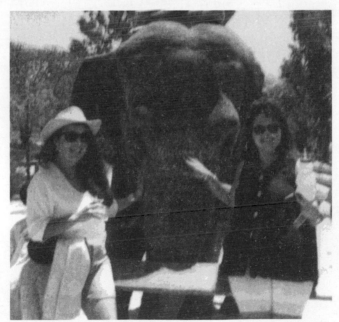

July 4, 1992, at Marine World Park, Vallejo, CA. Sylvia and Cynthia posing with elephant.

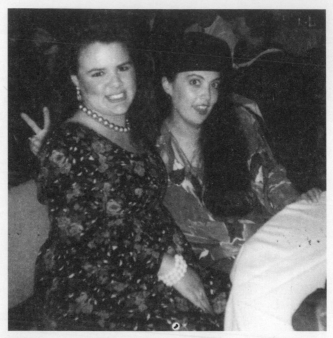

Cynthia and Sylvia at friend's wedding in October 1992. Note saucy beret Sylvia is wearing and the hand gesture she's making at Cynthia's back.

9

Sylvia's Transplanted Kidney
Shuts Down

In late summer of 1994, after returning home from the office, Cynthia called down from the upper level of our tri-level townhouse. She said that she'd just spoken to Terri on the telephone. The bad news was that Sylvia's kidney had reached the end of its transplanted life, and her body was rejecting it.

"Terri says she's back on dialysis, Mom." Cynthia remained at the railing. We exchanged a long, knowing look.

Rejection is perhaps the most feared word for transplant patients. For a kidney recipient it could initiate a severe condition called uremia, caused by accumulating toxins normally cleared through the body's elimination process. Because the kidneys are malfunctioning, these toxins are retained and literally poison the system. Dialysis is the artificial means of filtering the body's toxins by cleansing the blood. It confirmed that Sylvia's health was jeopardized, and her name would again be placed on the organ waiting list. At the time of her first surgery ten years earlier, the life expectancy of a transplanted kidney was between eleven and thirteen years. We cringed at realizing that the time had passed so quickly and that she was back on dialysis.

Cynthia's and my eyes reflected the emotions experienced in 1982 when we were shocked by Sylvia's sudden illness. My mind scrolled up the vivid memories of our *compadres'* kitchen table, where so many conversations about Sylvia's condition had taken place and how I had quizzed them: "So, what do the doctors say? How far up is she on the list? When do they think they'll have a match?" Those same questions would be voiced again.

Then, Maggie and Mando had wrestled with the dilemma of having Terri donate a kidney to her sister. Having one daughter in critical condition was bad enough, but to jeopardize their other daughter's life was too much to consider for any parent. Yet, as the months wore on, they felt they had no other choice but to accept Terri's offer. The fear of not finding a good match for Sylvia before it was too late became a looming threat. Terri unwaveringly stepped up to the plate, embracing the idea with a serenity beyond her years. I remembered so well the profound admiration she had stirred within us all. This time Terri had nothing left to donate.

I felt my face tighten as I recalled those worrisome months. In an effort to suppress them, I continued looking up at Cynthia. I watched in silence as she turned and went into her bedroom, leaving me to stare at the empty space she'd left behind.

In the compact kitchen, I plopped my purse down on the counter, poured a glass of ice water and went to stand before the living room window. The view was the reason I'd purchased the townhouse. To the east stood Mount Diablo, its dual peaks presented as one from our vantage point. In the foreground, San Francisco Bay's southern end glistened in the late summer sunlight as it made its way to Redwood Shores. It was a deep, royal blue today. Other days, it was gunmetal gray or light blue capped with white, feathery waves. On another afternoon it might be the shade of grayish sequins glinting in the sun. After a rainy or windy spell, it was muddy with brown swells. Whatever the color, its natural beauty always captivated me.

The San Mateo Bridge stretched from west to east, linking the Peninsula to the East Bay. The San Francisco International Airport busily received and dispatched aircraft. The vast stretch of highway known as 101 was filled with commuters. To the right, watershed hills greened the scene, creating a scenic delight that I never tire of and which never fails to soothe me after a tough day. Today, however, it offered little solace. Sadness veiled all within sight.

For the remainder of the evening, Cynthia stayed in her room, and I puttered aimlessly before going to bed. Even my old friend Agatha Christie couldn't hold my interest. I'm in the habit of rereading my collection of her books, working my way from *The ABC Murders* to Hercule Poirot's finale, *Curtain*, then starting over to repeat the sixty-odd-volume series again. Bestsellers are sandwiched in between, but Christie's whodunits remain my favorite escape.

Had I not been afraid of breaking down, I would've called Sylvia. It would be days before that happened. When I finally mustered the courage to call, Terri answered the phone and in a few words confirmed that we were in for a repeat of 1982.

Children have a way of surprising parents in the most unexpected ways. My twenty-four-year-old daughter was no exception. Shortly after learning about Sylvia's return to dialysis treatments, I arrived home from work to find Cynthia at the head of the stairs waiting for me. She greeted me with, "Mom, today I tested to see if I'm compatible to give Sylvia a kidney." A mixture of excitement, trepidation and pride shone from her face.

"What! You did what? How? Where?" I tried to hide my shock. How do you look supportive without betraying the inner alarm being triggered?

Fortunately, Cynthia was oblivious to it. She rushed to finish her news. "I went to Kaiser and took the preliminary blood tests. Boy, they took a lot of blood and…"

Her voice faded. I didn't hear the end of what she was saying because my own blood was pounding in my ears. Apprehension deafened me. All I could think of was, "Don't look afraid. Try and look proud. Don't betray the sense of love of family you've spent all these years fostering. Calm down. Easy."

When Cynthia is excited, she has a tendency to speak very fast, slurring her words so that sometimes I can't understand her. "Slow down, *mija*. Now, give it to me again."

I took her hand and led her to the sofa. "Sit. Tell me how you did this. Why didn't you mention it to me before?" I held back the questions popping into my head. I couldn't believe she'd done something so monumental without talking it over with me first. Being twenty-four years old didn't give her the right for such independent conduct, or so the mother in me thought.

She'd marched herself down to Kaiser and had the preliminary blood work done to determine if she was compatible with Sylvia and if her antibodies were well matched. An odd mixture of pride and anxiety overwhelmed me. Was I being hypocritical? *You want Cynthia and Joe to love family, yet you're getting hysterical when they do something to prove that love*, I told myself. The admiration I felt for my daughter at that moment was tempered by pain.

"*Mija*, are you sure you can do this? I mean, you're physically fit and everything?" *Shut up*, I told myself, *try not to rain on her parade.*

"Yep, the doctors first have to see the results of the tests. If they're okay, it looks like I'll be able to go ahead. It'll be about two weeks before I know the results." She beamed that killer smile the Zertuches are known for.

All I could do was give her a big hug and say, "Well, *mija, Dios dira.*"

Because I have a condition known as dry eyes, real tears have rarely flowed down my cheeks. In their place, I get a huge knot in my throat as if its function is to keep my heart from leaping out through my mouth. At that moment, I felt as though my throat was going to split.

Since it was Friday night, she was on her way out to visit friends. Popping up from the couch, she said, "I won't be too late, Mom. See you in the morning." She dashed upstairs, grabbed her suitcase of a purse, and headed for the door, jangling her keys on the way to the garage—spirit and feet floating. As soon as I heard the garage door close, I headed for the refrigerator for a glass of white wine.

I remained on the couch for awhile—paralyzed, not thinking or reacting—possibly, at times, not even breathing. History was repeating itself. One daughter saving the other daughter. I didn't know whether to rejoice, cry or pray. By the end of the evening, I'd end up doing all three. Was this how Maggie and Mando had felt eleven years ago?

How many times had Maggie jokingly said, "*Comadre*, why don't you take Sylvia and leave me with Cynthia? She's more like your daughter than mine and Cynthia is more like mine than yours."

It made us laugh while we recognized the germ of truth those words held. Cynthia adores her Tia Maggie, and I sincerely feel that Sylvia and I shared the same type of relationship. Keeping that in mind might make my dilemma more understandable. I had my daughter putting herself on the line for her cousin who was more like a sister; and, at the same time, my near-daughter was in desperate need of a kidney. In that light, Cynthia's decision seemed the way to go.

But what if Cynthia wasn't compatible? Sylvia's getting a kidney from the donor's list could take too long. The average waiting period was now up to four years. And if she wasn't strong enough, she might not be considered a good candidate for an organ donation. What then? I knew only too well what then. Sylvia's health would steadily decline, and she would die.

By this time, I was on my second glass of Gewurztraminer, my favorite wine. The verisol shades in the living room were still up, and the green scenery of late afternoon had darkened to shadows bisected by the freeway. Down below, speeding autos left red ribbons of movement in the southern direction, and white headlights streamed north. Runways from San Francisco International Airport were lit with orange lights. Airplane after airplane descended over Coyote Point to ease safely onto the runways at the water's edge. San Bruno's light standards caught the mist descending on the town in a ghostly luminescence. Beyond the bay, I knew that Fremont and Hayward awaited the return of their residents from the daily grind. Right now there would be an endless procession of cars on the San Mateo Bridge. I knew these things from memory, because at the moment, I stared out the window without seeing.

By the end of that evening a simple solution had revealed itself, an epiphany of sorts. Everything just fell into place. I had no feelings of nervousness or any qualms. It was as predictable as Terri's decision must have been, and I wasted no more time fretting about what might happen if Cynthia didn't qualify as a donor.

I was healthy. I hiked with the Sierra Club on weekends for up to ten miles and walked on the nearby three-mile Crystal Springs Trail several times during the week after work. I was full of energy. Why not me? I could do it. And Sylvia wouldn't be at the mercy of waiting her turn on the organ waiting list. And that's how it happened that within hours after Cynthia's announcement that she wanted to be Sylvia's donor, I became determined to take her place. Sylvia would get her kidney from me if it turned out that Cynthia was incompatible.

That night I said an extra prayer that one of us might be Sylvia's donor, and, as has been the case many times throughout my life, He answered it.

10

My Birthday Gift

The decision to give Sylvia a kidney might seem like a big decision in some people's eyes, but to me, it was one of the easiest things I'd ever done. To observe a loved one suffering from a failing organ is difficult, especially if that someone is barely thirty years of age. I had two of something that I only needed one of, and Sylvia had a deteriorating one that she'd received from Terri eleven years earlier. It was now worn out. Consequently, my niece and godchild was back on dialysis, back on a long, long list of prospective organ recipients, and back to carefully allocating lowered levels of precious energy in piecemeal fashion. For a vibrant young woman, it was a chokehold. For those of us who loved her, it was heart-wrenching.

Once Cynthia, terribly crestfallen, informed me that she'd been eliminated because she was incompatible, I told her of my decision to go through the requisite testing myself. It was thrilling to finally say it out loud. My heart pounded right into my throat, and hearing my own words filled me with excitement.

"Don't worry, it's okay, *mija*. I'm going to test."

It was Cynthia's turn to be silent, a rather rare response. She probably experienced the same thoughts I'd had when she told me of her plan to donate. Like me, she was adroit at camouflaging them. The announcement instantly snapped her out of the deep disappointment she felt at being rejected, and she gave me a huge bear hug. We were both so elated about the prospect that Sylvia could still be saved that we practically danced around the living room.

Inwardly, I suspected she, too, had the same misgivings about my going under the knife as I had had for her. She may have thought that, after all, I was fifty-three years old, a prehistoric specimen to those in their twenties. Doubts about whether I'd be acceptable as a donor probably weighed in. Whatever her thoughts, she kept them to herself. Once our euphoria subsided, I asked her for the name of the transplant coordinator at UCSF and promised her I'd get on it as soon as possible.

Because I've a superstition that telling anyone of an anticipated windfall or beneficial event might jinx it, I told her not to tell anyone else of my decision until we knew for certain that my being a donor was possible. I didn't want to get anyone's hopes up prematurely. Did she listen to me? No. Sheepishly, she confessed the following night that she'd been so excited about Sylvia's still getting a kidney that she simply couldn't keep from calling Terri.

"I'm sorry, Mom. I just couldn't help telling Terri about it."

I'm not so sure she was sorry, but before I could scold her, she slammed me with Terri's reaction. "Mom, when I told her, she didn't miss a beat before saying, 'Forget it, Sylvia will never let her do it. No way. Not in a million years.' And I think she's right."

I felt like I'd been hit by a two-by-four. That had never occurred to me. But I could picture Sylvia saying such a thing. I decided to shrug it off. "We'll see, *mija*. Sylvia's always listened to me before. Let's get the results first, then I'll deal with that issue."

Cynthia's raised eyebrows spoke volumes. Another moment of silence passed between us. Of course, it made sense: Sylvia wouldn't want to put me through major surgery. I totally understood Terri's statement. That was exactly what I would say in Sylvia's place. Why hadn't I anticipated it?

"I don't know, Mom. She's as stubborn as you are." Cynthia interrupted my train of thought.

I played down the importance of Terri's comment. "We'll see, *mija*. So, how about having some dinner?"

96

Deception isn't my style, especially with those I love. But, confronted with Sylvia's anticipated reaction, I must admit I toyed with incorporating deception into this current situation. Perhaps I could donate anonymously? Did Sylvia have to know who her donor was? How was I going to get Sylvia to allow me to give her my kidney? Actually, I would have tried trickery if I'd been convinced it would work. Shoving the dilemma aside, I went ahead with my original plan to be tested. But it continued nagging me all during my preliminary testing for donor compatibility.

My initial inquiry to the transplant coordinator at UCSF, Ana Marie, was enthusiastically received, and it seemed that I was placed on a fast track for the testing process. As Ana Marie explained to me, a factor equally as critical as blood compatibility was establishing that my antibodies would harmonize with Sylvia's antibodies. A thorough evaluation was needed to insure that both the donor's and the recipient's health wouldn't be jeopardized.

Ample assurances were given that at any stage I could change my mind, no questions asked. I knew in my mind, heart and soul that nothing could deter me. Even so, I truly appreciated the ethics practiced by UCSF's transplant unit in not pressuring me or making me feel guilty if I changed my mind. But would Sylvia herself derail me? That thought was an ever-present concern. Nevertheless, I started the process, hoping for positive results.

The first step was the blood tests. I arrived at the clinic in San Francisco at the appointed time, entered the cubicle where blood drawing takes place, and sat in a very comfortable, recliner-type chair. The technician asked me to roll up my blouse sleeve. I turned my face toward the wall to avoid seeing the needle. I don't mind being pricked if I don't see it coming. Observing my blood is a bit uncomfortable for me, even if it doesn't hurt.

As the technician tied the tourniquet around my upper arm, I turned my head back and nonchalantly said, "I understand you're taking ten vials today."

"Oh, no. I need more than that. Twelve ought to do it."

"Can I afford that much?" I blurted out.

"No problem. We do it all the time. Actually, it's not so much, maybe a bit under a pint. You can afford it. Are you the recipient or the donor?"

"The donor." The needle was expertly inserted after the usual words that there'd be a slight stinging sensation. After a while, I ventured a look at his handiwork. I watched as vial after vial filled, admiring my blood's gorgeous color. His touch was light and skillful as he slipped one vial in after another.

"Well, that's pretty nice. Still, you can afford a kidney. It's not like an eye. In the news last night I heard about a brother who donated one of his eyes to his other brother who'd lost the sight in both eyes after an accident. Now, that's something! Boy, that really impressed me."

"That's pretty impressive, all right," I said. "But I'm so near-sighted I couldn't give my eyes away, so I guess a kidney will have to do." I'd meant to be funny, but got no reaction.

As each tiny container was filled, it was placed upright in a metal container specially designed to hold the narrow glass tubes.

"Just two more to go," he said. When finished, he instructed, "Okay, keep this bandage on for an hour or so and apply a bit of pressure for about five minutes. That's it, all done." He snapped the tourniquet off, gathered up his blood collection and left with a nod and smile.

A few days later, the spot on my arm that had been injected with the needle bruised a bit. After the usual bluing, greening and yellowing, there was nothing to show for the experience. The following week, I was scheduled to leave on a week's vacation. I tried not to think about the results, which were due in approximately two weeks. Trying to squelch thoughts wasn't that easy. Since there was nothing to be done but wait, it was just as well I did go on vacation. When I returned from a short cruise to the Bahamas, I called Ana Marie and received great news.

"Well, Bel, you match in three categories. You have the same blood type, you've the same ethnic background, which helps, and your antibodies are in sync with Sylvia's. According to the blood tests, it looks like you are a possible donor." Ana Marie Torres' tone was businesslike, no emotion, except for what I perceived might be a hint of anticipation. Was she holding her breath, thinking I might have changed my mind? The ball had definitely been volleyed into my court.

I'd been holding my own breath and released it with a sigh. My first thought was, "Thank God," which was promptly followed by an audible, "So, what now? What's next?"

She started to say something, then cut it short to inquire, "Have you discussed this with Sylvia yet?"

"Uh, no. She doesn't know I've had the blood tests yet. I didn't want to get her hopes up in case I was incompatible, plus I'm afraid she might refuse my offer." I might as well come clean, I thought. "That's my biggest fear. Her sister doesn't think she'll let me do it. Is it possible to donate anonymously?"

In retrospect, it's incredible I could have had such a thought. My only excuse is that it seemed an easy solution. It was certainly much simpler and less demoralizing than losing the argument with Sylvia.

Ana Marie was quick with a resounding, "No! You HAVE to discuss this with her. There's no way we can proceed until you do."

"You mean I need her permission?" So much for my subterfuge scheme.

"Absolutely. And we'll need to have it before we go any further."

There's a psychological evaluation that's conducted with all prospective donors. I suspected I had just flunked it. Procedures had to be followed, and her reaction made all the sense in the world. We ended the conversation with my agreeing that she was one hundred percent correct and that I would approach the subject with Sylvia as soon as possible and get back to her.

As preposterous as it now sounds (and I'm usually quite level-headed), I had concocted a couple of scenarios whereby I'd give my kidney on an anonymous basis. In my desire to be Sylvia's donor, I rationalized that just giving her my kidney outweighed any objections she might have. I simply didn't want to give her an opportunity to refuse me. Her health, in my off-kilter mind, far outweighed common sense. As is frequently the case when trying to convince yourself you're right, you find ways to shuffle facts to your own advantage. The fact was, I was so fright-ened that I wouldn't be allowed to proceed that my thinking got skewed.

I wished with all my heart that somehow I could be her anonymous donor. It's awkward to confess these thoughts, especially since writing them down points out how nonsensical they were. But that's how desper-ate I was to avoid Sylvia's possible refusal.

I had the blood tests in September and received the results early in October. That was when I had my last conversation with Ana Marie. I pondered how and when I'd approach Sylvia. For two weeks I thought about it, discarding one approach in favor of another and yet another. I practiced speeches, mentally rehearsing possible lines of attack. I wrestled with what would produce the desired result of convincing Sylvia to accept my kidney. It was now autumn, and my birthday was around the corner, on November fifth. Sylvia never forgot my birthday, and I knew that therein lay the key to solving my problem.

Cynthia was aware of the blood test results and of the difficulty the next step entailed. Several times we sat on her bed exchanging ideas, though she didn't hold much hope for success. She squelched a few ideas with a simple, "Oh, Mom, puleese!" The fact that she was a tough audi-ence made her a good sounding board. She's definitely not a "yes" per-son. I threw out more possibilities.

"I'll give her a call and tell her I'm going up to Stockton to visit her on Sunday. We'll go out for brunch or something. Yes, at a restaurant so she can't get up and walk away. I'll ease into it. Say that I've looked into it, taken the tests and it'll work. She may object at first, but I think I can talk her into it and…"

Sympathetic though Cynthia is, she interrupted. "Mom, don't you think she'll think it's fishy popping up like that? It's not like Stockton is just down the street or anything. She'll know something's up. Nope, Terri's right. She's not going to let you do it, Mom. Face it."

She patted me on the knee, trying not to look too condescending.

"That's what you think, chickie," I replied. "Anyway, it's my birth-day the Saturday before that Sunday, and she usually makes it a point to see me then. So I'll just tell her that I know she's not feeling too well and

I've got the time to take a ride up. I'll make it sound natural enough. After all, it's been a while since I've seen her."

"I don't know, Mom. Don't get your hopes up."

Sometimes it's amusing when your children get to the stage where they think they know more than you do. I suspected Cynthia had arrived at that point when she became a teenager and had been lovingly humoring me for the last decade. Other times it's not so amusing. Especially if there's a sting of truth in what they say. She and I are lucky to have a relationship that is sensitive to each other's emotions. Different personalities don't often develop such a tight bond. It's a cherished link that I'm grateful to share with my daughter. It's uncanny sometimes how she can know me better than I know myself. It's that insight that made me sense she had an accurate read on Sylvia's reaction. Back to the drawing board, I thought.

Still unsure of how I'd approach Sylvia, I knew this weekend had to be the deadline. It was toward the end of October, and it just couldn't wait any longer. Sunday night I picked up the telephone and called her.

"Hi, *mija*, how are you?"

She always responded with "fine," although I knew from Terri's reports to Cynthia that she was on dialysis regularly, on Prednisone and feeling sluggish again. She managed a lift to her voice.

"That's good, *mija*. Say, we haven't seen each other for a couple of months, and I thought I'd take a run up next Sunday morning. Maybe we can have breakfast together. Just us. Somewhere like Marie Callender's or a favorite brunch place you might have. What do you think?" I hoped I wasn't talking too fast.

"Oh, that sounds great, *nina*. It'll be nice to see you."

She sounded sleepy, a side effect I recognized.

"Super. How's nine-thirty sound? I'll pick you up and we'll play it by ear."

"Just great, *nina*. I'll expect you then. How cool," Sylvia's melodious voice whispered through the phone line.

"Okay, see you then. In the meantime, take care, *mija*."

"Always, *nina*."

"Right. Love ya. Bye."

I hung up the phone, fighting my dry tears.

My throat thickened as I said a silent prayer for inspiration. That night, I started smoking again after quitting a few months earlier. It started with one cigarette in the evening, then two, but didn't go beyond that. When this is over, I told myself, I'll quit for good. In the meantime, the addictive crutch calmed my nerves. Still, it was an indulgence I wasn't proud of.

During the week I pondered ways I might bring up my proposal during our brunch. Scenes played round and round in my head. A tough approach? Should I beg? No, neither she nor I could swallow that. What would prevent her from saying no? What would prompt her to say yes? As I worked at my daily office routine, I kept searching for the most effective strategy.

Thursday of that week I called out to Cynthia as I returned from work. "Hi, *mija*. I'm home."

"Hi, Mom." She was standing in her usual place. "Terri called me today, and she's coming down with Gilbert on Saturday. He has to pick up a car or something. When Sylvia found out, she said she'd come down with her and save you the trip of going up on Sunday. They should be here about four in the afternoon." Cynthia's keen eyes watched for my reaction.

I needed a moment to think. My four sisters and I have birthdays within eight days of each other, from October 23rd to November 5th, and we had planned our usual birthday luncheon for that coming Saturday. Cynthia was aware of this, as she and Joe would naturally be there.

"Sure, we should be home by then. It'll work. When you call her back, tell her it's fine."

"Okay, Mom. So, what's for dinner?"

The Saturday birthday bash was great fun. We five sisters, one brother, spouses and children plus a couple of their friends had a wonderful luncheon at an allegedly haunted restaurant on Moss Beach, right on the edge of the Pacific Ocean. Our reserved room's back wall was an expanse of windows that showcased the beauty of the ever-changing sea.

It glistened gray on that fall day, as befitted the spirit of the Blue Lady. She is said to wander the pebbly beach below the restaurant. The ocean shone from the shore to the horizon. Waves foamed against the craggy rocks. Gulls squawked belligerently, and an occasional pelican skimmed the surf.

We ate amid a cacophony of conversations, laughter and camera flashes. The luncheon was a good distraction from worrying about talking to Sylvia. It ended about three-thirty, and by four we were home. On the drive back I'd thought of nothing else but my approach to Sylvia.

This was November of 1994, and for two years I'd been engaged to Don, a wonderful man who shared all that was going on in my life. We'd met on a Sierra Club walk after I'd been divorced seven years. He'd been divorced for four years. One of the things I did to keep busy on weekends was join the Sierra Club for hikes and walks. It was a great way to enjoy the beauty of nature and the camaraderie of a good group of people. Cynthia was twenty, and while we enjoyed each other's company at home, fun time was separate. Her social activity centered around her own friends, as it should have.

One Sunday in August of 1992, I met the Sierra Club Singles for a historic walk through the waterside town of Benicia on the Carquinez Strait in Solano County. The group gathered early in the morning, and as usual, the leaders had us introduce ourselves before describing the route we were covering. One of the newcomers was someone I hadn't seen before. Don Rennels was five feet eleven, with smiling blue eyes and a touch of shyness about him. I can remember wondering what an attractive man like him was doing running around loose. "Oh well," I thought. "He won't last long."

At some point during our town tour, Don edged up beside me and we fell into easy conversation. When the walk was over we all said our goodbyes and left. The following Thursday evening Don called me at home. I asked how he knew my phone number, and he said he'd looked it up in the phone book. A few days later he called again and we went out on an afternoon date. Before I knew it, we were seeing each other every weekend. Two and half months later, he proposed. Having him in my life at this time was a Godsend. It was especially comforting on this day. Knowing both he and Cynthia would be with me later boosted my courage.

Cynthia, Don and I sat around the townhouse and waited impatiently. I still wasn't sure what I was going to say. Just as Don and I were about to leave for five o'clock Mass, the doorbell rang and Cynthia hurried from the couch to answer it. In walked the noisy duo, Terri and Sylvia. As usual, the three greeted each other with feigned insults.

"Hi, *fea*" (ugly in Spanish), "what's up?" Terri let out her cackling laugh.

"Don't let her talk to you that way, Cindy. That's my job." Sylvia giggled.

As Terri and Cynthia tried to out-race each other up the stairs, Terri stumbled. Cynthia yelled, "Hey, wish I could be graceful," and slapped Terri on her backside as she edged ahead.

Sylvia trailed behind, shaking her head. I noticed her slower pace. Even though she was smiling, there was a tiredness about her.

Terri reached me first and gave me a big hug. "Hi, *tía*. How are you? Oh, yeah, and happy birthday."

I returned Terri's hug. "Thanks, *mija*. Fine, and you?"

Sylvia walked toward Don with outstretched arms for a hello hug. Then she turned to me. "*Nina*, happy birthday." I got an enthusiastic embrace and kiss. Returning her hug gave me the opportunity to shield the horrible ache of seeing the Prednisone's effects. Despite its necessity, the tell-tale bloated face and heavier body reinforced the urgency at hand. Mentally, I always conjure up her graduation picture, which hangs in my downstairs hallway to this day. Even now, underneath the chubbiness of her face, I only saw the beautiful sculpted features with their fine chin line, high cheekbones, perfect smile and dancing eyes that seemed to say, "Watch out, world, here I come." No matter what, I always saw beneath the puffiness to see her as she should have been.

I loosened from her embrace and said to both girls, "Don and I were just on our way to five o'clock Mass at St. Veronica's. You'll be here when I get back, right?" It was more of a request than a question. "There's plenty of goodies in the fridge, so don't leave, okay?"

"Sure, *nina*," Terri said, eyes bright. "We'll be here giving the brat a bad time. She's had it good for too long."

Cynthia snapped back with a tart remark in keeping with their habit of honing their wits on each other.

Turning to Terri, I asked, "Have you had dinner yet?" She shook her head. "Then I'll bring something back, okay? Maybe Chinese. See you in a little bit." With that, Don and I were out the door.

"You know they'll be talking a mile a minute all the time we're gone," I told Don, who, having had four sons, was not used to how girls interacted.

Don had been with me throughout the day and knew, along with Cynthia, that I planned to approach Sylvia that evening with my petition. He, as always, was being tremendously supportive, despite any misgivings he might have had about my submitting to major surgery. As we drove toward South City, he squeezed my hand. Funny how that small gesture is capable of transferring strength and support; I've grown to appreciate that touch a great deal.

During Mass I sought inspiration, but none seemed forthcoming. During the petitions, when the congregation responds "Lord, hear our prayers," I silently added my own plea for guidance. Finally, I decided to simply trust in God to help me choose the right words to convince Sylvia. Once leaving the matter in His hands, I relaxed. When Mass was over, we didn't dawdle at the front entrance of the vestibule to chat with old parish acquaintances. We simply left and headed straight for the car.

After picking up some Chinese food, we returned to the townhouse loaded with chow mein, beef and broccoli, almond chicken, moo-shu vegetables and fried rice. The girls weren't home. My first thought was that they were too hungry to wait for us and had gone out to get something on their own. But no, that was too out of character for them. Not knowing where they were made me nervous.

"I hope they heard me when I said we were picking something up for dinner," I told Don, who was carefully taking the styrofoam containers out of the plastic bags. As I grabbed plates and napkins, the telephone rang. It was Cynthia.

"Where are you?" I tried not to sound too anxious.

"We're at Cost Plus. Terri needed a coffee mug for her office, but we're on our way back. Be there in five minutes."

"Oh, good. We've got Chinese here. Hurry home."

"On our way. Bye, Mom."

I relayed the conversation to Don. He poured us a glass of wine, which I sipped while setting the table. Ten minutes later the door banged open and the loudest trio of cousins this side of the Mississippi stomped up the stairs. Sylvia was saying, "I told them not to be late, *nina*. But do they listen? No! You know how they are." She was smiling and pleased with her role as the self-appointed goody-two-shoes. Her cheeks were flushed and she seemed excited as she plopped down on one of the living room club chairs. I was pleased at how much she was enjoying herself, but couldn't help notice she was a bit out of breath.

"It's Terri's fault," Cynthia said, mostly out of habit.

"*Tia*, I needed the right mug for my desk, one with the right saying on it. We didn't think we'd be this long," Terri giggled in her high-pitched voice without any sign of remorse as she pulled out a garish mug from its bag. It looked big enough to hold a pint of anything.

"*Mija*, it's… well, it ought to hold plenty of whatever you want, that's for sure." I laughed. "Right. So, now you've got the right mug and we've got a cold dinner. Sit already."

Cynthia and Terri tossed off their sweat jackets and were in the kitchen surveying the cartons of food. Sylvia joined them. "Hey, leave me some." Each took whatever they wanted and zapped their plates in the microwave.

Don and I had filled our plates and were waiting for everyone to be seated. Finally, after much fussing we were all at the table. The girls kept popping up and down for refills, or a forgotten glass, or more soy sauce while Don and I watched, amused. I couldn't taste anything I ate. Much too soon, we were all finished eating. I noticed Sylvia's appetite wasn't at its usual level.

106

When fortune cookie predictions littered the table, I knew it was time. Sylvia was in the middle of asking about the birthday luncheon and I told her who was there, what we ate, how pretty the ocean looked. Then I popped out with, "Let me show you my cards and what I got. Some of them are pretty vicious." They knew what I meant by the word vicious. My sisters and I, as well as my two best friends, Kate and Kitty, try to buy each other cards that are unsentimental. Our taste runs to the sarcastic style of Shoebox cards that feature that old lady making cutting references about old age. We look for them all year round to make sure we've picked up the ones with the most biting humor.

I took my plate into the kitchen and headed downstairs to the den and my bedroom. Sylvia followed. We sat on my bed. She read a couple of the more vicious cards (my favorites) and seemed almost too happy. Was the medication affecting her? I showed her a couple of small gifts I'd received and she "aahed" at them. Eventually, I ran out of cards and presents.

"*Mija*, you know that today is my birthday?" I said.

She gave me a puzzled look. "Of course, *nina*. And I hope you're having a good one and many more to come."

"Yes, I am, *mija*. But there's one more thing I want, and only you can give it to me."

Her eyes widened, the smile vanished. "What, *nina*? You can have anything I have, you know that."

"Promise?"

"Yes. Anything, *nina*." She was fidgeting and obviously perplexed.

"Good, because I'm going to hold you to that promise. Remember what you've just said. You promised."

She nodded.

"I need you to let me do something." I kept my words coming, not wanting to give her a chance to interrupt. I took her hand in mine.

"I need you to let me give you a kidney."

There. It was out. "I've already been tested, and although we're not a perfect match, my blood type is right, our antibodies won't kill each other, and I'm a good candidate, *mija*. I've talked with your transplant coordinator, Ana Marie, and she says it's possible, although I still have to go through some final testing. But, *mija*, the additional testing is for me, not you. They want to make sure I'm in excellent health and that the quality of my life won't be diminished by having the one kidney. Then they'll X-ray my kidneys, insert a dye into me, take pictures so that you get the cutest one and…" That was as far as I got.

"Oh, no, *nina*. That's too much. I can't let you do that." She covered her face with both hands as she cried. She cried so hard the bed shook.

I steeled myself. "You promised!" I placed my hands firmly on her shoulders and inched closer until our thighs scrunched together. "Listen to me, *mija*. I'm not afraid. Do you think I'd put Joe or Cynthia or Don through something that would endanger my life? I'm in great health. I hike for miles, my blood pressure is fabulous. I'm never sick. Let me do this, please. We'll be fine."

I took her damp hands into mine. "I have a great deal of faith in God that he'll watch over us. I'm not afraid, *mija*, believe me. I know what it's like because I watched you and Terri go through it eleven years ago. We can have that same success again. Besides, you give my kidney two Hershey Kisses every night and it'll never know it's somewhere else."

That got me a giggle. After a moment, she said, "Oh, I have a lot of faith, too, *nina*, really I do." And I knew she meant it. "But I'd feel awful if anything happened…"

"Not to worry. I'm willing to leave it in His hands, how about you? It's really up to Him, isn't it? Remember, you promised me. God's in the driver's seat on this one, and I'm confident all will go well."

With an enormous bear hug and more tears, she managed to say that magic word, "Yes."

She dried her tears. I was so relieved. I could feel myself grinning. She went back up the stairs, with me close behind, and announced, "Guess what? *Nina's* giving me a kidney!"

Terri and Cynthia were speechless, and the looks on their faces were priceless. I detected a sense of resignation on Don's face, half enthusiastic and half apprehensive. While Sylvia and I were having our talk downstairs, Terri had asked him, "Do you know what she wants to talk to Sylvia about?" Don simply nodded. He's a man of few words, but much love and emotion. I did feel pangs of guilt for putting him and my children through this worry, yet they knew how critical it was for Sylvia and how important it was to me. Their courage in standing by me meant the world to me. Their support strengthened my resolve to be as healthy as I possibly could, and for their sake, to recuperate as quickly as possible. To that I was committed. In the meantime, we were all hugging.

Terri's face now looked softer, which brought home the realization of just how much stress she'd been under. She had wanted Sylvia to have a donor. But she was fearful Sylvia wouldn't allow me to be the one. I can only imagine how hard it must have been for her to see her sister deteriorate on a daily basis, to see the lethargy set in, the forgetfulness. Witnessing her decline had to be frightening, not knowing how fast or how far her debilitation would progress before she became incapacitated. How much longer could she work? Her salary contribution lightened Terri's financial responsibility, and although that was a secondary issue, it was a reality that would have to be dealt with. Hope oozed from Terri as she asked, "How about the blood tests, *tia*?"

"*Mija*, all taken care of. Unless I have some rare disease or the X-rays show something weird, it's a done deal. Now that I've got Sylvia's blessing, I can go through the remainder of the tests and then, ta da! Transplant time." I gave her another hug.

Cynthia was also elated. I made a mental note to talk to her later and reassure her that all would really go well. Joe, too, would need reassurance. But that would come later. For the moment I wanted to savor my victory, for that's what I considered this moment to be, a major triumph. That was Sylvia's special gift to me on that birthday—the most special gift I'll ever receive.

11

Surgery Is Scheduled

The following Monday morning, I could hardly wait to call UCSF's transplant coordinator's office. "Ana Marie? Sylvia says it's okay." I was laughing. "I'd like to get on with the rest of the testing as soon as possible."

"That's fine. Umm, let me talk to Sylvia first, and then we'll decide how to proceed."

I knew she needed Sylvia's confirmation. I gave her Sylvia's work number and asked that she call me back after they both had talked. About two hours later, a more animated Ana Marie called. "Where would you like to do the testing? Here, or at Kaiser in South San Francisco?" I opted for South City.

Linda, Ana Marie's assistant, wrote a detailed letter to Nurse Practitioner Moore at the Kaiser facility in South City specifying the different tests I needed to undergo. About a week later, I went in to see Nurse Moore. It was a welcome relief to find that all the requisite laboratory forms were already filled out. She spoke to me very briefly, asked some general health questions and pointed me in the direction of the laboratory. Such efficiency always impresses me, and I was grateful to get such quick action. That way, my time away from work was minimized, making it less stressful on my boss.

The lab work included lung X-rays, EKG, blood drawing and another urine specimen. A twenty-four hour urine collection regimen was also required, and I received a container with instructions for that analysis. The lab work was completed in a little over an hour. That night, when I called Sylvia to let her know I had done all this lab work, we laughed at the twenty-four hour urine collection.

"I didn't know I'd have to cart this pee container to work. When I leave in the morning, I have to make sure I take my pee cup. Maybe I should've borrowed Terri's new mug."

"Oh, *nina.*" Sylvia's giggle was getting softer, a dark reminder of our need for speed to complete the testing process.

Lab results took about two weeks, which is really pretty good timing. Still, who doesn't wish for instant results? This lull fostered silly (in retrospect) thoughts. What if I had some rare blood disease? I had once had a heart murmur, but that had disappeared when I reached my thirties. Would it matter if it came back? Maybe there was a spot on my lungs from when I used to smoke.

Was my urine all right? Thinking so much about my urine was certainly a novelty. Normally, it's such a routine, uneventful bodily process that you never give it any thought, forgetting how vital it is to maintaining good health. Now, self-esteem was linked to acceptance of my urine, and I caught myself staring at the toilet bowl each time I went. Was it the right color? I'd never noticed the different hues urine possesses before, and while it may seem gross to think about, I monitored my urine closely. This obsession with urinating took on a comic aspect. During our frequent telephone conversations, I talked about it with my sisters and we all laughed about it a lot.

The first order of business on the Monday after getting Sylvia's consent was to tell my boss, John, about the impending surgery and subsequent five to six weeks' absence from work needed to recuperate. After hearing this, he leaned his six-foot, heavy frame back in the reclining office chair and looked out the window at Richardson's Bay. Our office at that time was located in Mill Valley. It was his habit to look out at the water whenever he was thinking. He pondered for what seemed minutes, but I'm sure was only seconds. The more he objected to something, the longer this thoughtful stare took. The time always gave me an accurate gauge of what to expect.

"Bel, are you sure you can do this? You're not jeopardizing your health, are you? I can understand how you'd want to help Sylvia, but kid, let's be practical." At fifty-four, being called a kid at this juncture in my life was amusing.

"John, I'm fine. It'll be okay. You only need one kidney to function. My remaining kidney is going to get slightly larger and will do the job of two kidneys in a very short period of time. Remember, Terri hasn't had any problems at all having only one kidney. The transplant unit at UCSF has been super cautious about making sure I'm up to it. Not to worry. Also, I've called Linda, and she'll be able to be here in January and February."

John was a sixty-eight year-old bachelor, set in his ways, and he preferred smooth sailing, both metaphorically and in life. He loved fishing from his thirty four-foot boat and had sailed around the bay for many years. He was one of the founding partners of a large San Francisco accounting firm, Muncy, McPherson, McCune & Dieckman. He was the Dieckman and was now retired from the firm. After my previous boss, Decker G. McAllister, honorary chairman and founder of Pacific Scientific Company, died, John had become the vast estate's trust administrator. It was a natural transition, as John had been handling Mr. McAllister's accounting and tax needs for decades and was a very trusted friend of the McAllisters. For years our offices had been in Burlingame in order to be close to Hillsborough, where the widow lived. Once Mrs. McAllister died, John moved us closer to his Sausalito home. "Now it's your turn to commute," he said.

As his executive assistant, I was the only other employee in our office except for Linda, our part-time accountant who came in once a month. John was an exceptional steward. When I think of him, the word integrity looms in my mind. He was portly, very distinguished looking and well respected in the financial community. He depended on me to run the office, force the cantankerous machine known as the computer to spit out the required reports, and take care of any business contingencies that sometimes occurred.

Since smooth sailing in all aspects of his life was so important to him, he hated my absence from the office. I could never take more than two weeks' vacation even after ten years with the trust. Finally, in 1994, he relented and gave me an extra week as long as I promised not to take more than two weeks consecutively. Unfortunately, the office would close before I could enjoy that benefit. He died suddenly of a massive heart attack six and a half months after my surgery.

He was generous as far as my salary went, and every day that he was in the office, usually Monday through Thursday, we went to lunch together. It was his main meal of the day, and he hated eating alone. When he remodeled his kitchen and bathroom, I worked with the contractor, picking out the flooring, paint colors and bathroom accessories. In these areas, John was totally lost. Put him behind the wheel of a massive boat or place a pencil in his hand to crunch numbers, and he was a genius. Interior design, computers and office management were beyond his capacity or willingness to deal with. We were a good business team with deep mutual respect for each other. I shared my family life with him, and he routinely asked me about Joe, Cynthia and my sisters. I knew his concern about my surgery was genuine and tried again to ease his mind. I also felt compelled to convince him of my resolve and confidence.

"John, everything's fine. I'm in great health, the match is right. Sylvia and I will zip in the day before surgery, get it done and I'll be back home within five or six days. They say it'll take four to five weeks before I can come back to work, but Linda can sub for me, and she'll do fine. You know I'll leave everything up to date and oodles of notes for Linda. Plus, you or she can call me anytime once I'm home. Don't worry, it'll be fine. And you know what? I'm not at all apprehensive about it. Can't wait for it to happen."

His brows were still furrowed as he toyed with the ever-present pencil on his desk blotter.

"John," I reminded him, "do you know what will happen if she doesn't get a kidney soon?"

His gaze returned to the wildlife refuge waters. Finally, he said, "Yeah." With a deep sigh of capitulation, he added, "Well, I guess you've made up your mind."

The feminine mind seemed to baffle John, and he gave me one of his "What in the world are you doing?" looks. In this instance, his concern touched me. We'd been thrust together over ten years ago, and since that time we had worked hand in glove. In the process, a great deal of respect had solidified our working relationship. His great sense of humor made going to work fun; his expertise made it professional. I'd become fond of John and concerned about his well-being, just as I knew he was for mine. My announcement had probably broadsided him. It was the last thing he'd expected.

Eventually he became comfortable with having Linda fill in for me. I hadn't received the results from Kaiser or UCSF, so I wasn't sure what the time frame was. I promised to keep Linda posted. She graciously agreed to make herself available and was the first person to tell me what a good thing I was doing. That struck an odd note with me. Not that I didn't appreciate it, but being praised for being a donor was displeasing for some reason. If you saw someone drowning, wouldn't you jump in to save him or call for help? Praise seemed unwarranted, until I tried to see it from other people's points of view. Still, it made me uncomfortable to be commended.

I asked Linda and John not to mention the surgery to anyone else. Not that I was ashamed of it. It just seemed a natural act, so natural that it should not be deemed extraordinary. That's what I felt at the time. Today, I'm eager to talk about it in the hope of encouraging others who have a loved one suffering from kidney failure to consider being a donor. If people could see how unaffected I was by the nephrectomy, it might help lessen their own concerns.

I set about completing the qualification process. As much as I hate being a pest, I'm afraid that's exactly what I must have seemed to Ana Marie. Every few days I called her to see if the results from Kaiser were in. At the end of ten days, she suggested I call Kaiser directly. I did just that. Nurse Moore swore she'd mailed them out the previous Friday and couldn't understand why they hadn't been received. I called Ana Marie back, asking if she'd looked everywhere for the results and relating what Nurse Moore had told me. Poor Ana Marie must have been tired of hearing my voice. Eventually, the long-awaited results arrived at UCSF a week after being sent by Kaiser. And, wouldn't you know it, the twenty-four hour urine collection had to be redone.

Really, this preoccupation with urine had climbed to new heights. Or was something wrong with the results? Another thing to worry about. Carting around a plastic gallon jug and a collection funnel during working hours was comical the first time, not so funny the second time. I again dragged out my Nordstrom shopping bag, stuffed it with colorful tissue to camouflage the plastic jug, and carried it in and out of the restroom as nonchalantly as possible. On the day that I completed the second testing, I called Sylvia to update her on where I was in the approval process and couldn't help commenting, "Every time I pee now, I think of you, *mija.*"

We laughed. But even as we laughed, worrying thoughts filled my mind. Cynthia did a super job of keeping me posted on Sylvia's condition from her regular conversations with Terri. I learned that Sylvia was now on dialysis three times a week and having problems with sudden weight gain and forgetfulness. In addition, she was getting moodier.

Throughout her ordeal, Sylvia never complained to me or anyone else that I knew of. Such a silent, valiant effort on her part made the wait even more frustrating. For her mother, sister and brother it must have been doubly difficult to see her worsening each day. She was experiencing the emotional sensitivity and languidity symptomatic of patients undergoing kidney rejection, and every day became a trial for her and the family.

Sylvia and I were both aware that once the preliminary lab tests were evaluated and, hopefully, I passed muster, there remained two more critical tests to be scheduled. One was the crucial kidney examination, called an arteriogram, where a dye is injected into main arteries so that the surgeon can carefully scrutinize each kidney, compare the positions of the organs and, ultimately, decide which one to extract. Getting to that stage meant surgery was just around the corner. It was close, yet just beyond reach, or so it seemed at the time.

The single, most horrible thought plaguing me during this entire waiting period was the fear that something would prevent my being a donor; that Sylvia's hopes, as well as our family's and friends', would be shattered. And I can't imagine how I would have reacted or felt had the green light not been given. This consuming dread was exactly the reason for my wanting to do all the testing procedures anonymously. The thought that anything might interfere with the surgery terrified me. At times I felt confident that we were progressing, and I mentally prepared myself for being admitted into the hospital. Other times, doubts and uncertainties overwhelmed me and I was sure of nothing.

The UCSF doctors and staff had repeatedly advised me that I was a good match. Despite these assurances, I found myself constantly battling dark shadows of impending disappointment. This while trying to look confident. What if I was rejected as a donor in the final stages? What if some last-minute health problem arose? What if my kidneys didn't photograph well when the dye was injected? That was absurd. But what if, what if, what if… As the days passed, I tried to keep as busy as possible.

We were now into December. The final results from the second urine collection test still hadn't been received by UCSF. I pressed the kidney transplant coordinator about it every other day.

"Do you have the latest results from Kaiser yet?"

"No, they haven't shown up, and I've been on the lookout for them." Ana Marie seemed as anxious as I was. "Let me give them a call and see what I can find out. I'll get back to you."

I gave her the Kaiser number to call and tried to concentrate on work. Later that afternoon, Ana Marie called me at the office. "Boy, getting through to the right department at Kaiser isn't easy. No one knew a nurse named Moore. I got transferred from Medical One to Medical Two to Medical Three. Thank God they don't have a Medical Four."

We both chuckled at that. "Finally, I got a hold of a sympathetic soul to look for test results in your medical file. It turns out the results are in the mail to me, so I should have them sometime this week. I'll let you know the minute they come in so we can schedule the IVP and the arteriogram." With a few final words of encouragement, she hung up.

Three more days passed before I called her again. "Anything yet?"

"No, I can't imagine where they're at. I'd try calling again, but it's impossible to get through to anyone with any real information. If only I could get in touch with Nurse Moore." Even the usually efficient Ana Marie was beginning to sound frustrated.

"Let me try," I offered.

Kaiser is a great place if you know how to get around its maze of departments. I had twenty years of experience doing just that. So, using my best businesslike voice, I picked up the phone and started with the first of what I knew would be several extension transfers. At last, I located Nurse Moore.

Noting the frustration in my voice, she said, "I'm sorry for the delay, but some of the blood and urine tests were very complicated and took longer than expected. Still, I did mail them to Ana Marie four days ago. I personally placed all the results into an envelope. She should have them any day now. Give it two more days, and if they're not there by then, ring me back."

I thanked her, but was careful to verify her direct phone number in case I should need it again, although I told her I hoped I wouldn't. She echoed the same hope. I left Ana Marie a voicemail message about finally locating Nurse Moore and alerted her to expect the envelope any day.

The next day, Ana Marie called. "I've got them! Give the doctors a chance to review everything—a couple of days—and I'll get back to you. Hang in there, it shouldn't be much longer before we know for sure."

I wasn't interested in "much longer." I wanted the big, "Yes, let's do it!"

Each day on arriving home, Cynthia interrogated me. "So, what's going on? Anything new?"

While the tiniest tidbit of progress was welcomed, I was still frustrated. "Now we've got another three days or so for the doctors to look at the results. Geez, it's taking so long!"

Cynthia's great at letting me vent, seeing beyond it to the emotion causing the stress. I knew the information we exchanged would be faithfully relayed to Terri in Stockton that evening. Of course, Terri had experienced this entire testing and approval process firsthand over eleven years ago, but I hadn't been privy to that series of hurdles. I reminded myself that she was only twenty-one at the time, and a renewed appreciation of her experience grew. Surely, I could wait three more days.

We were all on pins and needles. Two days later, Ana Marie called. Without preamble, she blurted out, "You'll have to check into the hospital for a full day for the next tests. You'll need to rest for at least six hours afterwards in a hospital room after the procedure to make sure you don't have any side effects from the injection. When do you want to schedule it?"

I was dumbfounded. All of a sudden, I had a million questions. "Now, explain these tests to me again." My heart was pounding.

Patiently, Ana Marie explained that the first test was a series of x-rays of my kidneys. Then a specialist would administer a solution via an IV and more x-rays would be taken to map the exact position of each kidney. The second test consisted of an injection of dye into the kidneys to examine the arterial circulation aspects to and from both kidneys. These procedures assisted the doctors in examining the circulatory access and egress to the kidneys so that reconstruction of the arterial connections for placement into the recipient could be planned. It also afforded them the opportunity to determine which of the two kidneys would be the better one to remove. This is, of course, my simplified version of the process, but I believe it's accurate.

Until now my concentration had been so preoccupied with qualifying as a donor that the medical science making this miracle happen was taken for granted. Obviously, they can't go in and just snip out an organ and plop it into a recipient. I felt foolish that I hadn't given that any thought. Connections and disconnections have to be reviewed, studied and plotted. Also, I'd not considered the question of which kidney was to be extracted. Naively, I thought I'd be asked if I had a preference. Frankly, none of the details of the actual surgery had crossed my mind. I was so anxious to get into the operating room that I hadn't given any thought to the transplant details.

A new respect and admiration for transplant nephrologists and their teams took hold. I knew that the nephrologists and the transplant team at UCSF were the best and performed hundreds of such surgeries a year. So from the start I was confident Sylvia and I were in good hands.

In the meantime, my sisters had spread the word within the family, something I'd asked them to wait on until I was certain that the surgery could go ahead. One of my brothers, Art, had called me early on in the pre-approval process. He's an ex-police officer and not prone to talking much. In fact, the rest of us call him our Joe Friday from the *Dragnet* television series. You know, the "Just the facts, ma'am" type. Apparently, one of our sisters had called him to tell him of my decision to be a living donor, and he quickly responded by making a rare telephone call to me.

"You know, that really shows love. Lots of people talk about it, but you're doing something about it."

The tone in his voice was as loving as I've ever heard it, and it touched me beyond words that he would call and share so openly. Getting two running sentences from him was also a new experience.

My ex-brother-in-law, Charlie Zertuche, who is married to my first cousin, Maria Elena, so is now my cousin-in-law, also demonstrated loving concern when he heard of my decision. He and Maria Elena, or Nen, dropped by the townhouse to see me. I think he was a bit nervous for me. I tried to allay his fears for both Sylvia and myself.

"Really, Char, I'm looking forward to it. Not nervous about it at all. God will see us through, I'm sure." In a moment of weakness, he kissed my forehead and gave me a hug. Normally, we teased each other.

My sisters undoubtedly chatted among themselves about the matter. The twins, Esther and Elvie, as well as the other two, Beatriz and Betty, kept close telephone contact with me and with each other and saw each other frequently. Any news, good or bad, was immediately relayed via telephone. Opinions and feelings were shared. In this case, they were very respectful of my decision and understood the motivation behind it.

They were also aware of Sylvia's and my relationship. If they were concerned, they kept it to themselves.

I distinctly remember when I first told Don that I was considering being Sylvia's donor. We were riding in the car on our way to visit friends in San Jose. At that time, we hadn't heard the results of Cynthia's preliminary blood tests. Her decision and Sylvia's predicament weighed heavily on my mind. As we traveled closer to Carol and John's place, I finally voiced what had been brewing within me for days.

"Hon, I've been thinking. If it turns out that Cynthia can't be a donor for Sylvia, then I want to do it." There! It was out in the open. As I spoke the words, I heard the definite commitment in them and was pleased.

I heard a sharp intake of breath. "Gee, hon, do you think you can?"

I glanced at him and quickly tried to counter what I perceived to be a worried look. "I think so. After all, I can hike eight to ten miles, I don't have any illnesses or adverse medical conditions. I think I'm in pretty good health. Of course, I'd have to go through the testing process, but I think I'd pass."

I touched his arm as he kept driving. "I'll be okay, hon, really I will."

There was no attempt to dissuade me, just the silent support I've grown to cherish. From start to finish, he was fully supportive. He and my children bore the brunt of worry that accompanies such surgery, but it was also their love that enabled me to progress with such calm. I'll always be indebted to them.

The time between being found compatible and convincing Sylvia to let me be her donor seemed an eternity, but really spanned about three weeks. Once the medical hurdles were conquered, the anticipation of resolving Sylvia's kidney failure electrified our lives. I'm sure that knowing her transplant surgery was around the corner helped her endure the debilitating effects of her kidney failure. According to Terri's telephone accounts to Cynthia, the expectation of restored health improved her mood swings and disposition. It certainly gave my *comadre* and Terri hopeful expectation to know that Sylvia's deteriorating condition would soon be reversed. After all, they were the ones who, on a daily basis, witnessed the effects of Sylvia's declining health and personally dealt with the consequences. In my opinion, they were the real heroes in this drama.

Christmas 1994 passed with the knowledge that the New Year would see Sylvia with a new kidney. Thus it was an especially spiritual time of thanksgiving for us. At times I sensed a pervasive fretful feeling from Cynthia, Joe, Don, my sisters, my brothers and the rest of our large family. While I felt guilty about putting them through the ordeal of worrying about me, I knew the end result would prove rewarding. I was truly thrilled, confident and eager, and I tried to convey these feelings. Those two weeks prior to entering the hospital were, for me, full of joyous anticipation. It was Sylvia's and my adventure, and I could hardly wait for it to begin.

My kids gave me a combination breakfast and writing tray and a bed jacket as Christmas gifts. Leave it to Cynthia to be that practical and thoughtful and for Joe to go along with his sister's impeccable choices. As a wise brother, he's always supported her judgment in the selection of gifts throughout their adult years. That holiday was, for me, an especially blessed one.

12

The Odyssey Begins

On December 29th, Cynthia drove me to UCSF Medical Center for my IVP and kidney arteriogram. It was very early in the morning, and as instructed, I hadn't had anything to eat or drink since the previous day. Even without my regular coffee jolt, I was pretty excited that the finish line was in sight. Sylvia and I had talked the previous evening, and for the first time in many months, there was a cheerfulness in her voice. Soon, I thought to myself, soon, she'll be her old self again.

Cynthia dropped me off at the circular driveway on Parnassus Avenue and went off to park the car in the garage across the street. She'd taken time off work to do this. She was beginning to worry me because she seemed to waver between joy, fear and impatience to have the surgery over. I tried to talk her into just dropping me off, assuring her that Don would be there in the afternoon to bring me home. I promised to call before leaving the hospital. She wasn't having it. Have I mentioned that she's stubborn?

While she parked, I entered and found out where I was supposed to go. We arrived at the correct office after navigating a maze of twists and turns. Cynthia was asked to stay in the waiting room while I was ushered into a large room with a special x-ray gurney centered in the middle of it. To the side of the room I could see the customary glass-encased cubicle where the technician hides out during the zapping moments. After being directed to a tiny stall, I was told to change into a hospital gown. I reentered the x-ray room attractively attired in the short, buttonless frock. I wondered who had designed these gowns.

The x-ray technician had returned to his cubicle and was checking his equipment. About the time I lifted myself onto the gurney, a woman in a white coat entered the room. She greeted me warmly and introduced herself as the doctor who was going to insert the IV into me. She was my first real contact, and I took an immediate liking to her. She was probably in her late thirties and slender. I have the strongest recollection of looking into the eyes of a very attractive woman who turned out to have the most comforting and efficient bedside manner.

After the niceties, she calmly said, "I'll be inserting a catheter into your arm. That permits us to avoid two separate pinpricks into the veins. It also allows a convenient site for the insertion of this IV and for the injection of the dye and mild sedative used for the kidney arteriogram. Any questions?"

She was the type of physician that you willingly entrust yourself to, and I was terribly impressed that I was getting a full-fledged doctor for this preliminary step. What a gentle touch this marvelous doctor possessed! If you've ever had an IV inserted, you might have experienced a less than able hand inserting the needle, resulting in multiple, uncomfortable jabbing attempts. Mine was a completely smooth process. One slight prick and the IV was properly installed. Not only was the usual stabbing absent, but her demeanor was so professional and so caring that I was quickly relaxed. Here, I recognized, was the beginning of a wonderful experience. With a comforting pat on my hand and a dazzling smile, she turned me over to the x-ray technician and left.

I lay back on the x-ray table while the technician darted back and forth to position me, take a picture, and caution me, "Don't move," all while hustling back and forth from behind the barrier window. He was very pleasant and kept apologizing while he worked, especially for the need to place a heavy-weighted apron on my abdomen for a final series of shots. As he explained, this weight assisted in flattening the kidneys somewhat to allow for additional clarity in x-raying their shape, position relative to one another, position relative to the ribcage, etc. The weight was heavy on my stomach, but it was certainly bearable. The further we got into the testing, the more intrigued I was by the process—and thankful that medical science had progressed so much. It was fascinating.

The table I was on tilted to an almost-upright position. The technician, still apologizing for the inconvenience and assuring me that we were almost finished, raised the table to a perpendicular angle so that I stood on the bottom ledge of it. At that point, the ponderous weight started to bother me, but as promised, it was soon over. The last x-ray had been taken, and he rushed over to relieve me of the heavy pressure, returning the table to its horizontal position.

"All done. Now, let's get up slowly. Remember, you've got an IV in you. No sharp turns." He gently guided my legs over the edge of the table in preparation for me to step down. He handed me a plastic sack containing my clothing, then lifted the IV bag connected to my wrist off its stand.

"You hold on to your gown with your other hand and I'll carry the bag for you down to surgery." He addressed me softly and gently, as if speaking to a child.

Unbeknownst to me at the time, Cynthia had somehow gotten to a window where she could look inside and watch the x-ray procedure. The technician and I were now passing through that small anteroom. As we faced each other, Cynthia started to cry, which drew a puzzled reaction from the poor technician, who told her, "They're only x-rays."

"I know, but that's my mom," she muttered and kept on sniffling. I was flabbergasted to see her there and didn't know what to say. Whatever did come out of my mouth was, hopefully, comforting. Since my hands were occupied, one holding my clothes and the other the hospital gown, I couldn't reach out to hug her. I felt awful about causing the tears and reassured her that everything was fine and would continue to be fine. It helped knowing that Cynthia, more than others, could appreciate the necessity of going through with whatever it took to help Sylvia.

"*Mija*, it's all right. It was nothing. They do this all the time. You go on now. By the time you get home from work, Don will call and let you know what time to expect me home. I'm going to be resting for six hours. How hard can that be? Give me a kiss and scoot." She dried her tears and attempted a brave smile. "Remember," I said, "this is for Sylvia. Call her and tell her everything's going along fine."

That produced a genuine smile, and with a quick peck to my cheek, she was off, leaving a frazzled technician in her wake. "My, she's very emotional, isn't she?"

I smiled. "Don't worry, you didn't make her cry. She's just a bit nervous, that's all."

He silently took me to the elevator, walked me downstairs to a surgery room, handed me over to a nurse and left. I think I thanked him as many times as he had apologized earlier.

The waiting nurse was tender and competent. She guided me and my IV pole to yet another table in the middle of a very large, white, stark room which looked more like a laboratory than a surgery. She assisted me onto the gurney. Anchored to the ceiling above it was a TV monitor.

She noticed me looking at it, smiled and said, "You can watch if you like."

Returning to the long work counter lining the opposite wall, she opened up a file and asked, "Have you been told about this next step?"

"Yes, I'm sure it was explained, but could you repeat it for me, please? I seem to be blanking out on some of the details."

She patiently described what was about to occur. "Well, the doctor is going to inject a dye into your main artery in the groin area…" As she continued, I remembered hearing the explanation before. The dye would make my kidneys visible for x-ray purposes so that their placement could be evaluated for the surgeon's scrutiny. After reviewing the pictures, they'd decide which kidney was the best candidate for transplantation. I could easily observe the television monitor from where I lay and was curious to see what I looked like from the inside.

Finishing her thorough explanation, the nurse went back to the counter and flipped through another file. Knowing what to expect is such a big help. Learning about each step and the reasoning behind it was of great importance to me. Patients usually fear the unknown more than the known, and the time she took to explain the procedure again had a soothing, reassuring effect.

Still looking through the file folder, she asked me some routine questions about age, if I smoked (I'd stopped before Thanksgiving), what kind of work I did, etc. Returning to take my blood pressure, she pointed again to the anchored television unit.

"I think you'll find looking at your kidneys interesting."

"Great. I promised Sylvia the cutest one. You know, I should've contacted a plastic surgeon and had a face lift and liposuction at the same time. Might as well, since I'll be recuperating from this anyway." I was half-serious.

"Oh, come on," she said. "You don't even look your age."

That may be the prescribed reply, but it works. "That's because I'm lying down. You should see me when I'm standing and gravity takes over."

We were chuckling when the doctor came in. He was rather young and got right down to business. The older I get, the younger everyone else seems to be—from doctors to baseball players to sales clerks.

He explained the procedure to me all over again. I appreciated his earnest approach, but really felt like just getting on with it. Describing the injection, he said, "You'll feel a warm sensation, you may even think you're urinating" (there's that word again), "but it's just the dye flowing through your system. If you feel strange, or as if you're going to pass out, let me know. Okay? Great. Let's get started."

Hooray, it was beginning! The injection felt like a slight prick, a sensation without discomfort. The anticipated warmth coursed through my lower body and was not unpleasant, just warming as he'd said. After a few moments, I looked up at the monitor and there was the inside of my body. What a mind-blowing trip to actually see inside yourself! I stared at my kidneys, the most prominent objects on the screen. They weren't at all kidney-shaped, as in a "kidney-shaped pool." Rather, they were an asymmetrical pair of elongated, misshapen ovals suspended on either side of my spine—more like pears. They also seemed misaligned, one being slightly higher than the other. This, I was told, is quite normal. Amazing!

I was looking *inside* me. Even though the background was gray and fuzzy, the sight of my innards on that monitor was so remarkable it kept my eyes glued to the screen.

After a few minutes, the doctor announced, "We're almost done."

When the time was up, he added, "Now, be very still while I apply pressure to the entry puncture. I'll need to do this for about ten minutes. You okay?"

"Fine, thank you, doctor."

I wanted to giggle at the sight of this handsome young physician standing over me pressing against my groin area for a full ten minutes. He looked as intent as if it were the most complicated task in the world, which I appreciated. Actually, everything seemed to carry humor that day.

He placed a dressing over the tiny puncture area, bid me good luck and goodbye, and was off. Then I was delivered upstairs to a patient room, where I was to lie absolutely flat and remain still for six hours. This is not an easy task, especially when you're feeling excited and not at all ill or sleepy. I still couldn't eat or drink. Obediently I lay still, but I couldn't wait to talk to Cynthia, who would then call Terri, who would then tell Sylvia and Maggie. At last, I thought, staring at the ceiling. At last.

About an hour and a half later, Don appeared in the room, bent over me and kissed my forehead. That really made me giggle. He'd never kissed me on the forehead before, and I thought it was so cute. More-over, it was such a strange experience to be lying flat in bed with a guard rail surrounding me and having him standing next to me. He actually looked different from that angle, although his blue eyes were as appealing as ever.

He held my hand as I described what had happened during the day and what a curious experience it was to see one's insides. Don is an engi-neer, which makes him curious about the workings of equipment, and he listened attentively. Since he'd traveled from his office in San Jose, I knew he'd probably missed lunch. I encouraged him to go down to the cafe-teria for a bite to eat. Satisfied that I was in fine spirits and things had gone well, he left.

"Take your time, hon. I'm not going anywhere." This got me another kiss on the forehead.

He'd just left when Ana Marie walked part way into the room. She beamed at me, looking very businesslike in her neat skirt and blouse and with clipboard in hand. At that moment, I knew it was truly a bona fide go. I burst out with a huge belly laugh, so thankful and so proud of my lopsided kidneys.

"Hey! Didn't I tell you I had killer kidneys? Didn't I?" I felt like an athlete who'd just made the Olympic team.

"Yep, it looks like a go, all right." Ana Marie was at the guard rail. "Everything looks good. When do you want to schedule surgery?"

"The sooner the better. Is Sylvia ready? Does she have any preparation to go through?" It suddenly occurred to me she might have some preliminary work that needed to be done.

"I think she is. I'll call her. But as far as I know, she's all set." She looked at a schedule attached to the clipboard "How about the fifth of January?"

Suddenly, things were really zipping along. "Uh, that just gives me two days at work after New Year's. I've got to get some year-end reports out and, with the holidays, that really doesn't give me enough time. Still, I don't want to postpone it. What's the soonest available date after the fifth?"

"Well, kidney surgery is done on Tuesdays and Thursdays. You have to come in a full day ahead of time for prep. How about Tuesday the tenth? You'll come in Monday the ninth." Her pencil was at the ready.

"If that's okay with Sylvia and her doctors, it's better. It'll give me four days at the office. Okay, let's set it up," I said.

Nodding, she twirled around and quickly left. She was back in fifteen minutes. "Sylvia says the tenth is fine. Looks like we're all set."

I couldn't quite interpret the expression on her face, but it was definitely full of emotion. It may have been a mixture of relief, satisfaction, efficiency, gratification. Whatever it was, I liked it. It gave me insight into her deep commitment to her profession. This wasn't just a job to her.

"Okay. Now, how about getting me out of here?" I asked. "How much longer do I have to stay?" Being still is not one of my strong points, and with the news of scheduling the date, it was getting tougher and tougher just to lie there.

"Let me check with the nurse. I'm off to get this paperwork started. Congratulations. I'll stop by and see both of you when you come in on the ninth." She was still aglow when she left.

Don returned a few minutes later. "I'm sorry you missed Ana Marie," I said. "She was just here, and guess what? It's okay. I can do it. Isn't that great? Do I have killer kidneys or what?"

"Hon, that's wonderful." I received another kiss on the forehead and it had the same effect as before. As I stifled a giggle, he took my hand, squeezed it and said, "I love you, babe." As with Cynthia, I detected a bit of apprehension.

"Everything's going to be all right, hon," I whispered as reassuringly as possible. "You'll see. I'm not worried, so don't you worry."

We called Cynthia to say that we'd be home in a couple of hours and gave her the surgery date. There was no need to ask her to call Terri. She promptly offered, "I'll call Terri and let her know, Mom." I didn't tell her that Sylvia had probably already told her and Maggie, because I knew she needed to talk to her cousins herself.

Eleven more days. What a way to start the New Year. There wasn't an iota of doubt in my mind that Sylvia's health was secure.

13

The Eve of Our Surgery

The day before Sylvia and I were to report to the hospital for pre-surgery testing, Terri and Sylvia drove from Stockton to the townhouse. This long-awaited day was the morning of Sunday, January eighth. Remarkably, not one of us talked much about the upcoming surgery, but instead concentrated on enjoying each other's company. The three cousins went out for a while, then came back and watched TV in Cynthia's room. I could hear an occasional laugh, a bit of teasing and subdued murmurings.

Sylvia's condition had, fortunately, not deteriorated greatly. Her lower energy level was still obvious, as was the swelling to her features caused by the Prednisone. The important factor was that she was still strong enough to undergo transplantation surgery. Her outlook was positive, and whatever symptoms might be plaguing her, she kept them to herself. I knew the girls were concentrating on enjoying every moment. Any nervousness was covered by laughter.

At seven o'clock that evening, Terri left our place to return home, as she had to work the next morning. My *comadre* would be at the hospital on Tuesday, and depending on the outcome, Terri might drive down after work. Since Sylvia wasn't working, Terri's paycheck was vital to pay the bills. Just as Sylvia never complained about her condition, Terri never complained about the pressures as breadwinner. She bore that commitment with as much courage and grace as Sylvia bore her illness.

At seven-thirty a.m. on Monday, January ninth, Cynthia delivered Sylvia and me to UCSF Medical Center, dropped us off at the front door, and turned around to go back to South City's new Gateway Office complex, where she worked. Heavy rain pelted all of San Francisco, creating huge puddles and cascading down its famous hills. Sylvia and I, both in sweat suits, shook ourselves off and trotted into the admissions office to fill out the required forms.

A friend of mine, Alice Herrera, worked at the medical center and was aware that we were being admitted that morning. She and I had children the same ages; her son was my son's age and her daughter was my daughter's age. They'd attended St. Veronica's School in South City together, where Alice and I first met. Working together on some of the same school guild committees and attending the same school functions, we had developed a friendship and had kept in touch over the years.

Before Sylvia and I had finished our paperwork, Alice entered the waiting room, looking around. I rose to meet her hug.

She said, "Hi! I wondered what time you'd come in. I was going to call down about ten o'clock to see if you'd checked in yet, but decided just to pop in to let 'em know to call me when you arrived. When are you scheduled?"

"First thing tomorrow morning. Oh, by the way, this is Sylvia."

Sylvia nodded, smiled, said, "Hi, nice to meet you," and returned to filling out her form.

Turning to Alice, I said, "I've got a Dr. Juliet Melzer as surgeon. Ever hear of her? What's her rep? And Sylvia has a Dr. Peter Stock. What about him?"

"Both excellent, Bel. We've got top surgeons in nephrology. They really enjoy excellent reputations." She gave us a warm smile. "Well, I've got to get back to my desk. I'll stop by and see you later, after the testing is over. Okay?" On her way out, she tapped the desk counter to get the admissions clerk's attention. "Take good care of them." Alice then turned to wave goodbye to us and left.

The clerk looked up, smiling. "Of course." She quickly went back to work on the morass of paperwork spread in front of her. We completed and handed in our forms. She gave them a quick review before ordering us to present ourselves at the nursing station on our assigned floor. We each carried a small tote bag and were in great spirits. It was like following the Yellow Brick Road.

Sylvia and I were on the same floor, but assigned to different rooms. My room was surprisingly large. A generous expanse of window faced the Golden Gate Park Panhandle, and I could glimpse Sutro Tower through wafting steam from vents on the roof below. I liked the expanse of windows in the room. It was a cool, waterlogged day, and the air outside coated the windows with fat beads of water sliding down the glass. The inside was beginning to fog up, but not enough to block out the wide, green-zoned backdrop of dripping treetops in the park. Some paid many thousands of dollars for such a view, and here I was getting it for free. Life was good.

I changed from my sweats to the traditional blue hospital gown, threw on my comfy lounging robe from home, and placed the few toiletries I'd brought in my bed stand. A young nurse came in.

"Hi! I'm Barbara, and I'll be your nurse 'til afternoon. We'll have a few tests for you. Just a routine blood and urine sampling, an EKG, and a treadmill test."

I sat on the edge of the bed and automatically held out my arm as I watched Barbara take the blood pressure apparatus off the wall. My pressure was good, moderately low, as usual. She took my temperature, felt my pulse, wrote notes on the medical chart, and advised me that both Dr. Melzer and the anesthesiologist would be speaking to me sometime today.

"How are you feeling?" she asked.

"Excited. Terrific. Can't wait to get it over with."

"That's wonderful. If there's something you need, I'll be at the nurse's desk. You can walk around if you like; stay close, though. They'll be looking to give you an EKG and the other tests I mentioned."

I found out that Sylvia's room was about four rooms to the right of the corridor and headed that way.

"Hi, *mija*," I said, smiling at the nurse beside her. I looked around her room. "This is just like mine. Bigger than I expected. Did they tell you we're going to get visits from the surgeons and anesthesiologists? So I guess we can't sneak down to the cafeteria."

Sylvia acknowledged me with a little smile. I settled onto her bed, where she sat upright, leaning against the pillows. The rolling food tray was tucked in front of Sylvia, and she was going through the medications in what looked like a fishing tackle box. The nurse silently accepted each medication as Sylvia named it and handed it over. There were so many dosages to keep track of that she needed more than the normal pill containers. The quantity of different containers astounded me. Sylvia expertly examined each compartment of the box, flipping one bottle aside, counting pills in another, saying the name of each medication out loud, ticking it off verbally to her nurse. Finally, she closed the lid and relinquished the box to the nurse. "Yep, I think that's it. Everything seems to be there."

The nurse thanked her and whisked the meds away.

The sight of all those medications tugged at my heartstrings. It was great consolation to know that, after tomorrow, it would be different.

"Oh, *nina*, I'm so hungry." Sylvia pushed aside the tray. "I'm all up to date with my medicines. This afternoon I'll go in for dialysis. I wonder what time we'll see the doctors?" Her color was good, I thought, and her voice full of hope.

"I don't know, but I'm getting pretty hungry myself." We were both on a liquid diet until early afternoon. After that, there'd be nothing, not even water.

"Wouldn't a chocolate milkshake taste good?" I said.

She gave me the famous Sylvia giggle. "Ay, *nina*, stop that."

Just then the anesthesiologist rapped on the open door. "Hello. I'm looking for Bel Zertuche. She's not in her room."

"That's me. Is it okay to talk here?" I remained stretched across the foot of the bed.

"Oh, sure. This'll be fine," the anesthesiologist said. He walked around the bed and sat down on the chair against the window. His pale green surgical garb made him look rather casual and young. The concerned voice and compassion in his eyes were instantly comforting. As he explained his role and the various surgery stages involved, I knew I could rely on him.

"How long do you think we'll be out?" I asked for both of us, even though Sylvia would have her own anesthesiologist.

"Five hours or so, maybe less. I'll be checking you very carefully during all that time, so don't worry."

"One thing that's really important to me," I said, looking directly into his eyes for emphasis. "I'd like to be completely out before entering the operating room. I don't want to see any equipment, utensils or overhead lights. Is that possible?" I had this dramatic picture in my head from old movies of a cold operating room, huge overhead lights and masked doctors surrounding the patient. Then came the loud music, rising to a crescendo, tightening my nerves before the screen faded. I didn't want any reminders of that type of scene.

"No problem. We'll slip you something in pre-op." He smiled, patted me on my leg and said, to my embarrassment, "You're doing a great thing, and we're going to take very good care of you."

His compliment threw me. I didn't want any praise and simply said, "Thank you."

Sylvia, on the other hand, eagerly volunteered, "Yes, she sure is."

He left, and we were like two little kids on Christmas Eve. We talked about nothing and chuckled about everything. Nurses popped in occasionally to check in on us and relay some bit of information. "The physical therapist will be around soon." Or, "We need some more blood." Or, "Let's check that blood pressure." We each had our turn.

I felt like I was on a vacation and savored playing hooky from the office. It was especially joyful because of the reason for my absence. Overall, I was flying high when Dr. Juliet Melzer strode in.

"Oh, here you are. I've been looking for you." Her gifted hands were slipped into the white coat that identified her as a doctor.

The instant her voice reached my ears, I knew that God had sent me the right person. She was very businesslike as she sat on the chair beside Sylvia's bed. She spoke directly to me, aware that Sylvia was listening. I was still reclined on Sylvia's bed, facing Dr. Melzer and listening intently. She explained in great detail every aspect of the next morning's operation. I urged my brain to absorb as much as possible.

"We've decided to take the right kidney since it hangs lower. We won't have to break a rib with that choice."

That was news to me. No one had mentioned having a rib broken. I tried to hide my surprise.

"You're going to be positioned on your left side, arms stretched upwards like this." Her approximately five-foot, six inch frame rose momentarily to give me a live demonstration of the position. Her arm was raised as high as it would go. Pointing to her waist area, she said, "You'll be stretched out like this, which gives us better access to the kidney. It's not just a matter of snipping it out, you know. We've got to carefully disconnect the arteries, which is why the IVP and arteriogram testing was so important. It showed us the circulatory paths to and from the kidney. As soon as we take it out it will be placed on ice, in a container, for speedy transport to Sylvia's doctor. He'll have her ready for the implant. You'll be in twin operating rooms, of course."

She looked at Sylvia. "Your doctor, Dr. Peter Stock, will have prepared you for the transplant by this time."

Back to me. "I'll close you off. Make sure everything's fine. There'll be multiple layers to sew up, about five. The inner stitches will dissolve eventually on their own. The top layer will be taped with paper strips."

"Paper tape?" I blurted. That didn't strike me as being adequate.

"Yes, it works fine. We squeeze the skin together like this." She pinched a part of her forearm. "Tape it together and it works very well. The whole thing should take about five hours. Afterwards, you'll be returned to post-op, then your room."

To my surprise, she added, "You won't have anything to drink or eat for about three days." Her voice and demeanor turned stern. "Now, it's very important that you not drink anything or eat anything for that period of time. You have to understand that your system will be completely shut down for five hours or more, and until we can hear evidence from your stomach that it's reactivating on its own, you can't have a drop or morsel. Clear?"

"Evidence?"

"Gurgling sounds. Rumblings from your stomach and your intestines."

"Oh." I looked at Sylvia and raised my eyebrows. Not eating for three days was going to be a real challenge.

Sylvia watched me the whole time Dr. Melzer was speaking. Was she looking for fear, doubt, regret? If so, I know she didn't find them.

"Any questions?" Dr. Melzer said, leaning back and crossing her legs. She wore no makeup. Her skin was flawless. She had short, glossy, dark hair and a contrasting pale complexion that reminded me of Snow White. Her eyes might have been hazel. It's amazing that I can't remember for sure, because they were aimed so piercingly at me. She'd given me an intelligent, no-nonsense description of the surgery. It was so detailed and to the point, I couldn't think of anything else to ask.

Then I remembered. "I asked the anesthesiologist not to let me see the operating room or any of the lights or surgical instruments."

"No problem, I'm sure he'll see to it," she said.

"Also, I'm concerned about the pain when I come out of the anesthetic. I'd like whatever pain medication I can take and enough of it to keep me comfortable. I'm not in the habit of taking pills, but I'd like whatever you can give me."

Dr. Melzer nodded and relaxed a little, softening her professional edge. "Well, what I can do is give you a button on your IV. This'll release a shot of morphine whenever you zap it. It's a regulated amount, naturally, but you administer it to yourself as you need it. Say, before you get up to go to the bathroom. Or if you're feeling a greater degree of discomfort. It seems to work quite well. And, of course, you'll be on other pain medications as needed."

I felt reassured. "Sounds good to me, doctor."

I didn't have any more questions, and she didn't dawdle. "See you in the morning then." She got up and left.

"I like her," I told Sylvia, who already knew it from reading me so intently.

"Yeah, she seems pretty nice—and smart, too. I like my doctor, too." She rearranged herself on the bed before asking, "You nervous, *nina*?"

I'd been waiting for that. "*Mija*, I can't wait to get it done and over with. If I had a do-it-yourself kit, I'd do it myself."

"Ay, *nina*." And she giggled.

My response seemed to relax her. We lounged around a bit longer before my nurse came to fetch me back to my room.

"Time to insert the IV. Got to keep those liquids flowing to the kidneys, you know."

I was back on my bed. "A hydrated kidney is a happy kidney," the nurse said as she hooked up the bag to its portable pole. She examined my arm and hand. "Let's see how your veins are." She rolled her finger-tips around my wrist and lower arm area. "My, you have a lot of valves."

"Valves? What are those?"

"Well, they're a little like lids that flip back and forth to aid the cir-culation to the heart. I can feel them all along here." She continued ex-amining for just the right spot to prick, lightly fingering the area around my hands and wrist. "Yes, I think this one will do." She took a large needle from her smock.

The first attempt at injecting the IV needle was difficult. "What tough veins! I can't get through properly." Her brows came together as she concentrated on her task. I flinched in response to a couple of fruit-less efforts. The IV injection during my previous tests had gone so smoothly that I hadn't anticipated this type of problem. Nobody wants to be surprised when hospitalized. I tried to maintain my composure. Then she gave up.

"I'm sorry, I'll have to try again." She rubbed my upper wrist sooth-ingly, as if trying to make amends for the unsuccessful invasions. "You okay?"

"Oh, sure," I said, trying to act nonchalant.

"I'll let you take a little breather." Her fingers began searching for a fresh entry spot. A couple of minutes later, she said, "All right, let's try here. It feels like a good spot."

She rubbed it spot with a damp cotton ball and pierced me again. No good. My stoicism was slipping fast. No matter how hard she tried, the needle refused to puncture properly—either that, or my veins were like rubber. I couldn't imagine why this IV was being so darn difficult.

The nurse finally gave up and withdrew the needle. "I'm so sorry," she said. "I'll let you a rest for a while, then we'll have to try again. We've got to get those liquids in you."

I wasn't disappointed to see her leave. Not wanting to just sit there, I went back to Sylvia's room. "Well, no luck." I managed a laugh. "Either I've got thick skin, tough veins or a poor nurse. All of which means no IV. Not yet, anyway. She'll be back later. Don't you just hate those things, *mija*? I think they're the worst part of surgery." Sylvia had lots of experience with IVs and shunts.

Sylvia nodded. "Oh, I hate them, too. Sometimes you get someone who just slips them in so easily and you don't feel a thing. But when they don't have that magic touch, boy oh boy, can it hurt. Once, in dialysis, I had a nurse put a needle in wrong and there was blood all over the place. I had to yell after her and point it out to her. I was soooo mad that time."

I mentally kicked myself. Sylvia had more reasons to complain than I'd ever have in a lifetime. Every hour I became more and more aware of what kidney failure does to a person. With that awareness came a deeper love for this wonderful, cheerful, non-complaining young woman.

We surfed television channels but found nothing but talk shows and soap operas. Neither was of interest to us. Sylvia was dozing off. She was prone to do this at this stage of rejection. I picked up a *People Magazine* I'd brought with me and flipped through the pages. I just read the captions under the pictures because I couldn't concentrate on the articles. In a few minutes, the physical therapist came in.

"There you are. I'm about to start an exercise session down the hall. Want to join us?" She directed this inquiry to me.

"What kind of exercise?" I asked.

"Well, we do some therapy. That's for post-op patients, usually. But we also have a treadmill, and I think you should spend some time on that."

"Good, I love to walk. I'll do the treadmill."

Sylvia had awakened at the sound of another voice. The therapist asked her, "How about you? Interested?"

"I'm waiting to go into dialysis. Sorry," Sylvia replied with a sleepy grin.

"I'll catch you later, *mija*." I jumped up from my chair and followed the therapist down to the physical therapy room at the end of the hall.

I did about a half an hour on the treadmill, finding it harder than the regular walks I took several times a week. But the activity felt good. On my way back from the therapy room, I peeked into Sylvia's room. She wasn't there. I assumed she'd been whisked off to her dialysis session, so I returned to my room. Shortly, I was joined by my day nurse plus one more.

"Bel, Nancy is going to give you the IV." She'd obviously passed the baton to another teammate.

Nancy, in her professional tone, said, "Let's see what we have here." Barbara, I think, had been talking behind my back. Finding my arm to be quite ordinary, she concentrated on the hand and wrist areas. She chose a spot on the top of my hand, just below the wrist, dabbed it with alcohol and thrust in the needle. The confident look on her face turned to perplexity. She addressed her fellow nurse. "Wow, now I know what you meant." Looking at me, she said, "Your veins ARE tough."

I tried to keep from squirming as she probed with the needle. It hurt. Perspiration flecked her upper lip as she pushed the needle in further. I bit my lip and clenched my free hand. Finally, she stopped.

"I'm going to leave it here. It's not quite all the way in, but I'll tape it and I think it'll allow the flow-through. Maybe during surgery they can relocate it." She stared at the crooked needle jutting out of the top of my hand. With a sigh, she gathered up her things and left.

I might have thought it comical, except every time I moved, the IV smarted. I was at a loss to explain why the one on the day of testing had gone so smoothly and this one was so awkward. It would continue to irritate me until it was properly placed during the following day's surgery.

I went off to look for Sylvia. Talking with her would distract me from the misery in my hand. I rolled the IV stand along with me. A nurse directed me to the dialysis room, and I soon found myself peeking into a four-bed ward. Sylvia was in a recliner-type chair next to the window on the left, chatting with a technician. They were speaking dialysis lingo. Sylvia looked across at me as I entered. "This is my *nina*," she said with a smile.

I can't remember what the technician said. The sight of Sylvia on dialysis staggered me. I fought to appear calm and unaffected by the mechanics of keeping Sylvia alive. Blood was being extracted from her body through thick, clear plastic tubes connected to a boxy metal receptacle next to the chair. As this mechanical kidney filtered her blood, other tubes on the opposite side returned the cleansed blood to where it belonged. Her blood swooshed up and down, across her body. It circulated over and under the light bedcovering in the same type of plastic tubes, across to the other side and back into her body.

The apparatus repelled me. Instead of viewing it as the blessed, life-saving technique it is, I'm ashamed to admit it sickened me. I clenched my IV pole until I thought it would snap. Smiling away the lump in my throat, I murmured, "*Mija*, this is the last time." The words comforted me more than they did her.

Sylvia snapped back. "Yep. Hopefully, it is." She remained reclined and so very calm. This blood-laundering was, after all, an integral part of her life. Just as I brushed my teeth, she dialyzed. The difference was that if I didn't brush, I wouldn't die. That thought steadied me. I could start to appreciate just what a great gift dialysis is.

That scene cemented my resolve and summoned a heartfelt reverence for all that Sylvia endured as a patient with kidney failure. She'd told me earlier that the process took three to four hours, and the thought had made me dizzy. I leaned over and kissed her forehead. "I'm going back now and dream of my next juicy cheeseburger with loads of pickles.

Are you as hungry as I am?" I tried to sound lighthearted, and I think I got away with it.

"Not really, *nina*. Give me a couple more hours, though. Once I start watching TV, I know there'll be nothing but food ads and I'll start salivating." She rolled her eyes.

"My mind is doing that for me right now." I grabbed my IV pole and left.

Late in the afternoon, after Sylvia returned from dialysis and had awakened from a nap, I went back to her room. The television set was on, but her attention was on the magazine she was flipping through.

"Hi! I'm walking around as much as I can and thought I'd pop in to see you. How ya' doing?" My free hand was behind my back as I walked around her bed.

"I feel pretty good, *nina*. Isn't the time dragging!"

"It sure is. The food trays are working their way down the hall, and I can smell the food. It's driving me nuts." Actually, anticipating the impending surgery had squashed my appetite. I whipped out a cellophane package I was hiding behind my back and placed it on the bed tray in front of her.

"Kisses!" She yelled as she laughed. "Ay, *nina*, you and your Hershey Kisses."

"Remember what I told you the day you promised to let me be your donor? My kidney has to have Hershey Kisses every day or it might go into withdrawal. Two or three ought to do the trick, but you can't skip a day. Normally, I have them at night while I'm in bed reading. Don't forget." I leaned over and gave her a hug.

I got another, "Ay, *nina*." Returning the hug with a giant squeeze, she whispered, "Thank you so much, *nina*."

"Now don't get mushy on me. We can't waste H_2O on tears." I pecked her on the cheek and straightened up. "Got to go now. My night nurse is chomping at the bit to give me an enema. Boy, that was a surprise. If I'd known they had to do that, I might have changed my mind."

You'd think the prospect of major surgery couldn't be overshadowed by much. Try enema—the old-fashioned kind. No amount of

medical progress, new drugs, innovative technology or other break-
through had eliminated the necessity of applying that primitive tool. The
last time I'd seen a hot water bottle with its treacherous tubing was
when my daughter had been born over twenty years ago.

My night nurse was a formidable African-American woman whose
demeanor shouted professionalism and no nonsense. She was full-
figured without being fat, about five feet, four inches. The moment I saw
her, I knew there'd be no coddling from this nurse. But I found her
generous with her explanations of all the details involved in prepping me
for morning surgery. I felt thankful to be in such competent hands. She
examined my medical chart with such intensity I thought she was memo-
rizing it.

It was past seven. I'd asked Cynthia, Joe and Don not to visit that
evening, as I knew they were planning to be here the following day. I had
brief, cheery phone conversations with each and assured them I'd get a
good night's sleep. Tomorrow their own ordeal would also be over, and
that eased my conscience. Their apprehension had been the only regret
about my decision. I was particularly worried about Cynthia, whose tears
always cause me consternation.

Joe was a different type of worry. My twenty-nine-year-old son
tended to safeguard his feelings, shielding them from outward display—
at least from me. I had no idea what he really thought of this transplant
surgery. I did know that he was wanting success for Sylvia's sake. The day
I told him of my decision, he typically joked, "What if I need one?" This
was quickly followed by an embrace and, "I love you, Mom." I knew
Cynthia had probably snitched before I got to him, so he wasn't taken
completely off guard.

I encouraged him not to come to the hospital until the surgery
was over. "I'll be out of it anyway. If you're here when I wake up, that's
plenty, *mijo*. So do as you please, but don't feel you have to be here every
minute."

He gave me a "We'll see," and I dropped it.

I knew Cynthia and Don could not be dissuaded. They'd be at hand
from beginning to end, and I didn't even try to talk them out of it. Don's

staunch support fostered a serenity, and I was especially grateful to have him keep an eye on Cynthia for me.

By ten o'clock, my strict nurse had finished administering the dreaded series of enemas. This is not a graceful procedure. With all the medical advances and new technology, has no one come up with a better way to get this job done? I thought of that old song, "If My Friends Could See Me Now," from the Broadway show *Sweet Charity*, and was grateful no one could. I bore it with as much poise as could be mustered. In looking back, the memory makes me chuckle.

When it was all over, I finally relaxed with a bit of reading. Eventually, my nurse entered my room again, reread the chart, took my blood pressure, returned to the chart to make some notes, and softly asked, "Did they take a urine specimen from you today?"

"No, I don't think so. They said they would be, and they took lots of blood, but I didn't pee into a cup, if that's what you're asking."

"That's exactly what I mean. You're sure they didn't take a specimen?" Her voice rose with an odd firmness.

"I'm sure. The nurse got so involved with trying to insert the IV, I guess she forgot about the specimen."

The look on her face told me that she was expecting a sample. I immediately wondered if there was anything left to produce. "I don't think I've got anything else to give." I kept staring at her as she continued flipping through the pages in the chart.

After a few seconds, she said, "Nope, don't see it here. I'll be right back. Got to phone the lab."

Alarms went off in my mind. My normally calm nurse was noticeably troubled by the lack of a specimen. I knew how important it was to get my creatinine levels. It directly relates to the working efficiency of the kidneys, and they needed to be at the right levels to proceed. I began to panic. What if they postponed the surgery? Could they? Suddenly I remembered being in Sylvia's room when her nurse had entered carrying the tell-tale paper cup and requesting it be used. Why had I missed the fact that I hadn't received my container? How dumb! Damn, if it was postponed...

The last awful notion froze me up. I couldn't bear to think further than the beginning of that thought. Just then, my nurse returned. In her hand was a paper cup.

"See what you can do," she said. "The lab will run it through tonight in time for tomorrow. Let's get it to them right away. Just do what you can." She stood near the lavatory door. I promptly obeyed, greatly relieved there'd be no cancellation. Me and my shadow, the IV pole, reentered the bathroom. Success. I managed to provide enough for testing, which the nurse whisked away. The crisis was averted thanks to her attentive, quick actions. All systems were go, and zero hour was just hours away.

14

Mission Accomplished

I can't remember sleeping that night. I must have, because I do remember waking up. It was very early and all was quiet as I lay still, waiting for the start of the Great Moment. The gap between the draw drapes
revealed a repeat of yesterday's weather. Rain was already pelting against
the panes. Mini-cascades trickled and slid down to puddle on the case-
ment. It was about six o'clock in the morning, and I felt oddly heavy
even though I was lying down. The night nurse was still on duty. Nurses
were working longer shifts and fewer days, or so I'd heard, because of the
economy. My nurse was reading the medical binder again. She must have
had it memorized by now.

Was that me whimpering? I couldn't believe it. I hate crying because I do it so poorly. Since I have dry eyes, tears don't well up to pour
over my cheeks. They don't spill out dramatically as proof of my heart-
wrenching inner spasms. Instead, tearless, staccato-like sobs overtake
me, and they can be awkward and embarrassing. I couldn't believe my
lack of self-control.

The nurse tried to comfort me. "Oh, that's all right, honey. Just a
little anxiety attack, that's all. You'll be okay, you'll see." She patted my
hand as she strapped the blood pressure wrap about my upper arm. "It's
going to be over before you know it. I think they're on their way up
now."

"I know, I know. I just don't know what's the matter with me." I couldn't explain the crying jag. It wasn't because I was scared or nervous. In fact, it was too early for me to be thinking or feeling anything. I'm not a morning person.

"Sylvia, is she up?" I asked. The last thing in the world I wanted was to let her see me like this.

"Don't know. You're my case, but she's probably awake or will be soon. Let's just get you settled down. Oh, here they are."

"They" turned out to be one person. He and my nurse exchanged looks during the silent transfer of her responsibility. He took hold of my bed and started turning it about. She fussed a bit over me for a moment, straightening out the blankets and making me neat for my journey.

"I'll see you in a couple of days. I'm not working tomorrow. You're going to be fine. So, 'til then, take care and be good." Those words soothed me immensely. I heard her whisper to my driver, "She just had a little anxiety attack, but she's fine now."

He nodded as he wheeled me down the corridor to the special elevators reserved for patients. He smiled, said very little if anything, and delivered me through the double doors leading to the room they called pre-op. The tattle-tale snitched to the nurse in special operating garb who was waiting for me.

"She's had a little bit of a cry."

I covered my eyes to screen out the bright lights bombarding me so early in the morning. My driver placed me where instructed, in a space behind a circular curtain of blue. I could hear muted conversation. Someone was saying, "No, I couldn't get through, so I stayed at a friend's place. Hope I make it tonight."

Unusually heavy January rainstorms were creating havoc all over the Bay Area, especially with the roads. Commuters resorted to alternate means of getting to and from work, including staying with friends. Another voice was responding to a query: "No, she didn't make it. Roads closed. They called the next one on the list. He'll get it."

Even in my state, I knew what that meant. Someone on the organ transplant waiting list had been bumped due to bad weather and her inability to present herself quickly. I could only imagine the disappointment and heartache of the intended recipient—and the profound joy of the replacement whose turn had suddenly arrived.

What a quirk of fate. I was struck that something as natural as rain had altered two lives so drastically. The enormity of it all overwhelmed me. I felt helpless, vulnerable and anxious. I started crying again. I had gone years and years without crying, so this double occurrence unsettled me. There was no choice but to just let it run its course.

A young female nurse in a pale green wrap-around top and matching slacks approached. She leaned over and smiled. "The anesthesiologist will be here shortly to talk to you." She reached for a bag of fluid and expertly hooked it on to a bedside stand. Satisfied, she examined the hand where the IV was inserted. I winced as it moved.

"We'll get it in better during surgery." At that point, she noticed I'd been crying and said, "That's all right, everybody gets a little nervous. We'll be giving you a sedative soon. Not to worry."

I didn't respond because right then I heard Sylvia being wheeled into the space adjacent to mine. The dividing curtain between us was pushed back, and I had a clear view of her. As her gurney was positioned, I again noticed how swollen her features were due to the steroids.

Instantly, I stopped crying. She was groggy eyed, but I knew she was awake because she and her driver were talking quietly.

"Good morning, *mija*. You all right?"

In a slur of words, she mumbled, "Yeah, *nina*, but I'm so sleepy."

I was still looking over at her when the anesthesiologist poked through the curtain and stood at the side of my bed. He looked freshly scrubbed and perky. "Well, we're all set to go. It'll be soon."

I reminded him of my wish not to see the operating room, and he reassured me, "Not to worry. We're giving you a sedative in about two shakes. Everything will be fine."

He disappeared, and seconds later another nurse materialized. She approached the IV pole and did something to it, then turned to me. "Just a little bit of sedative and…"

The last thing I remember is looking toward her as she fiddled with the IV bag. The exact moment when my eyelids closed will always remain a mystery, for I sure don't remember shutting them…

My ears awoke first. I heard sounds of nurses coaxing Sylvia awake somewhere across from me as I came to. I wondered why she wasn't next to me. A frightening thought formed in my drowsy mind.

"Oh, my God! They forgot to take me in! She's back, it's over and I never went in." Somewhere in that burst of panic, logic fought for recognition. Then someone was tapping my feet and not giving me time to think properly.

A faraway voice chided, "Come on now, sleepy head. Time to go back up."

The tugging at my feet continued. Across the way, identical pleas were directed at Sylvia. "Time to go up now, come on, wake up."

I was in a whirl; nothing made sense. Of course, they wouldn't forget me, how silly. But four or five hours couldn't have elapsed—that kind of time doesn't go by in a blink of an eye, does it? The bed rolled away from the coolness of the post-op room. Were they taking me into the operating room? No, she'd said "upstairs." Everything was confusion. I ebbed in and out of being awake. I was deliciously adrift between consciousness and some tranquil space without boundaries. As I hovered in this carefree limbo, I succumbed to a lightness of being never experienced before.

Eventually, in one of my drifts, I noticed I was being steered down an endless hallway. Squeaking wheels led the way. The building seemed empty and silent except for the steady whining of my gurney. A tall, handsome man rushed toward me, his blue eyes scanning my face.

Even in my stupor, I noticed his hands in his pants pockets, jingling their contents—a nervous habit of his.

"Hi, honey," he said.

Cynthia's face emerged next to Don's. She'd been crying. A smile forced itself toward me. Despite my drowsiness, I knew it was over. We'd done it! I sank back into dreamland.

Cynthia and Don stayed with me as I slipped in and out of consciousness. I remember holding two precious hands against my bosom, squeezing them, because I knew they belonged to my daughter and Don. I felt a residual coldness from the recovery room and kept wondering where Sylvia was. Inexplicably, nothing mattered and everything mattered.

"Wake up, you sleepy head." It was my good friend Carol. Imagine, ultra-busy Carol taking time out to be here. She and her husband, John, owned a business in San Jose that took up most of their lives. Yet she was somewhere in the room, talking to Cynthia and Don. Joe swirled in the background. I heard him tell his sister he'd gotten a haircut earlier in the day. I sensed the enormity of Cynthia's silence and tried my best to smile up at her. "See, *mija*. I told you it would be okay."

Subconsciously I felt relieved that both sides of my family didn't have to worry about the surgery any more. My side, the Toscanos, had shown me a lot of support when we were together. I found out later that they did discuss some concerns privately. They couldn't help wondering if I'd be okay. And would the transplant be successful for Sylvia? They never let their anxiety show in my presence. But as soon as Cynthia called them to say that I was out of recovery, the telephone wires between their households hummed. And my brothers found out the results from "the girls," which has always been the routine.

It wasn't until years later, when I found out how they'd prayed for Sylvia and me, that I realized how tight-lipped they'd been about keeping their anxiety from me. It was appreciated almost as much as the prayers. Actually, both meant a lot to me.

The Zertuche side might have been less anxious because they remembered Terri's positive experience of eleven years earlier. On the other hand, I wasn't as young, so perhaps there was some concern. If so, they'd never let on. Their form of support was simply to be there. Sometime in the afternoon on the day of surgery, I recall my *comadre* and her sister walking into my room. She neared the bed, touched my hand and said, "*Gracias, comadre. Dios te bendiga*"(may God bless you). Then in English, she added, "You've done a wonderful thing for our Sylvia."

I don't know if I replied. She must have been at the hospital most of the day with Sylvia, both before and after the surgery. I can only imagine how extremely difficult it was for her to see her daughter go through surgery a second time. I was thrilled at the nephrectomy's success just as much for my *comadre*, Terri and Gil as I was for Sylvia. I truly felt the depth of Maggie's appreciation. It was not only heart-warming, but fulfilling.

Sensing my current painless state was temporary, I embraced it. I remember savoring it, not wanting it to end. Nonetheless, I heard myself ask, "Sylvia? How's Sylvia?" A voice informed me that she was fine.

Time was a blur, but I was conscious that my loved ones were there. I can't explain how much their presence comforted me. It permeated the air, giving me a feeling of security. At some point everyone left, probably more exhausted than I.

The doctors and nurses had told me prior to surgery that before the day was out, I'd be walking. Around eleven o'clock that night, the threat was carried out.

"Zap yourself," a new nurse instructed, pointing to the morphine button hooked onto my IV. I had Dr. Melzer to thank for that. I hadn't used it yet, but now I pressed the button.

Throughout the weeks, I'd wondered what waking up from the operation would be like. Would it be excruciatingly painful? I'd shoved that thought aside. I knew I'd be given pain medication as needed, and I can truthfully say that I didn't fret over it. Now I did.

I heard the lowering of the bed rails and tried to raise myself. Someone must have filled me with lead while they were extracting my kidney. My body was rigid and wouldn't maneuver. It simply wasn't obeying.

"Come on, easy does it." Her voice was tender but firm. "Swing your legs first, that's it. Let's get this around you." She placed a short robe around me, guiding my left arm through the sleeve. She draped the right side over my shoulder to accommodate the IV. I kept repeating, "Oh, oh." It wasn't painful, as I recall. There was just a feeling that my body didn't want to move, as if it would break.

I placed my elastic-stockinged feet onto the cold floor, but couldn't quite straighten up. It felt like I was riveted to the floor in a clumsy, hunched-over stance. Then it came. A dull pain. It grew, spreading through my body, brain and senses. I could hardly see. Didn't want to speak or move. Oddly, the actual incision around the waist didn't hurt. But my innards were extremely sore, raw from being probed. Fortunately, the morphine masked some of this. With the nurse's assistance, I shuffled toward the room's doorway.

"You need to walk," the nurse explained. "Just take it easy, you're doing okay." She was strong when I leaned heavily on her. I kept inching toward the door. The short distance seemed a block away.

Sylvia and I had made a bet: who could walk to the other one's room first? The wager was five dollars. At that moment, I had no illusions of winning.

When we reached the door, I peered around the corner to see a vast stretch of corridor. Blessedly, the nurse said, "That's enough for now. Let's turn, slowly. Good."

I hobbled back to the bed, exhausted. No one would believe that these wobbly legs were capable of hiking nine to twelve miles on a regular basis. My arm eagerly stretched forward to touch the rumpled covers. At last. I eased slowly back onto the bed and melded into the soft mattress. I sank into a blissful sleep.

A short time later, a powerful dryness roused me, and I rang for the nurse. Because I couldn't drink or eat for three days, she moistened my lips with a swab of glycerin. That did nothing to quench my thirst. But it did alleviate the stinging of my parched lips.

Hanging from the bedside was a urine collection bag that was routinely emptied, measured and tested for creatinine levels. A catheter had been inserted during surgery to facilitate voiding and to eliminate the necessity of having to get in and out of bed too often for a few days. Judging by the rate of production, the remaining kidney was doing a bang-up job. The fact that my remaining kidney was functioning so well was a very positive result. It was a much bigger yardstick than I realized at the time. Someone had said during the preliminary testing that one's remaining kidney simply takes over the job of both kidneys and, in fact, may become slightly larger in the process. How prudent of nature to instill this life-saving capability! My creatinine levels were also steadily achieving satisfactory readings.

This surgery phase may seem scary or appalling to some. I'm not trying to overemphasize it. In fact, the time passed so quickly that whatever pain I felt faded away. But one cannot undergo a donor nephrectomy without some pain. It's best to be realistic about that fact. Likewise, a root canal is not without pain, nor childbirth, nor heart surgery. Yet the results produce relief, happiness or an extended life. In this case, Sylvia's life was extended, and mine was fulfilled. Add to that the relief felt by Maggie, Terri, Gilbert, the rest of the family and all our friends. The small amount of pain I put up with was worth it a thousand fold.

As a donor, I can attest that I have experienced no negative consequences as a result of this surgery. More importantly, the satisfaction of having given Sylvia a chance for a normal life was worth it. Would I go through it again knowing about the post-operative effects? Absolutely, positively, resoundingly, "Yes!"

The following three days were a blur of white coats darting in and out, nurses frequently taking my blood pressure, needles drawing blood, and an acute thirst. UCSF Medical Center is a teaching hospital, and bands of white-frocked student doctors occasionally huddled over me. Before they entered any patient room, the students were briefed and cross-examined about the patient's symptoms, current status, and prognosis. I remember Dr. Melzer escorting a troop in to see me soon after my surgery. She examined my incision, changed the dressing and asked me to cough. The idea of coughing or sneezing was unwelcome, and I gave the weakest possible attempt.

"Come on, now," urged Dr. Melzer. "A brave lady like you can do better than that."

"Being brave is highly overrated," I muttered. I took a deep breath and gave it another try, wincing at the effort.

"Much better," she said as she pressed around the paper-taped wound and displayed my waist to the medical students. "No redness, looks clean. It's going to heal beautifully," she said, rightly pleased at her handiwork.

I couldn't bring myself to look at the incision even when I showered, which I was allowed to do on the second day. I was content to have the doctors and nurses inspect it without giving it a look myself. That feeling was perhaps irrational, but I had it and indulged it.

The second day I had visitors. Cynthia and my good friend Kitty were in the room sometime during the day. I could hear them chatting as I continued to fluctuate between sleep and semi-wakefulness. The buzz of their conversation and occasional giggles woke me up a couple of times. I think I asked them to quiet down once—nicely, I hope. I don't know how long they stayed, or if I had any other visitors that day.

The zapper button was getting frequent use. At one point, I opened my eyes and caught a glimpse of Sylvia walking by, turning my way, thinking me to be asleep and continuing on. "I owe her five bucks," I thought. Later, I learned she had ventured in to see me the day after surgery, but found me asleep. I think she was worried about my condition. She may even have felt a touch of guilt about it. She didn't return to my room until after I was able to visit her.

For the record, this surgery is harder on the donor than on the recipient. The reason, as explained to me, is that the impact of inserting a kidney into a recipient is not as intrusive to the body as is the extraction of the kidney from the donor. In 1995, an open nephrectomy, as mine was, resulted in an incision of approximately seven to eight inches along the side of the waist. This, in itself, contributed to the length of recuperative time. Also, in making the incision and the necessary artery connections, nerve endings were irritated. When a nerve is disturbed, the results can be felt at points further away from the area of contact. A jab on the left side of the body may be the result of a nerve irritation on the right side of the body.

The procedure has advanced considerably since our surgery in January of 1995. A lathroscopic nephrectomy, a much less intrusive procedure, is now available. The hospital stay currently is two to five days versus the seven to nine days of years ago. (See Dr. William Amend's interview, Chapter 23, describing these improvements.)

During the operation, my kidney, once inserted into Sylvia, had begun producing urine right on the operating table. For the recipient, there probably is no greater news than that. I confess to taking a sinful amount of pride in my little transplanted organ. All my fears about not being an effective donor were gone. It was doing its job for Sylvia. We couldn't ask for more.

One unexpected aspect of our hospitalization was the number of family and friends who visited us. Cousins, nieces, nephews, Sylvia's friends, my friends, my children's friends—all took time from their lives to share with us. Alice, the school friend who worked at the medical center, also dropped by to see me a couple of times. My room looked like a florist shop, and cards covered the windowsill. Sylvia also got her share. We were overwhelmed with attention, and it was a priceless compliment. I can say without equivocation: visiting a person in the hospital imparts a special feeling to the patient. It can't be measured, and it's never forgotten. During the days of our convalescence, Sylvia and I fondly recalled every person that came by while we were hospitalized. Their names became etched in our memories.

Cynthia, Joe and Don were frequent visitors during the days immediately after surgery. My brother Art, our Joe Friday, visited me twice: once when I was alone, and another time when Don was there. As he and Don talked, with an occasional word from me, I vividly remember enjoying listening to Art. I can't remember what he said, but it was the most I'd ever heard him talk. It delighted me. I was also flattered that he'd made the trek from Santa Rosa into the city, especially since I knew how much he detested driving into the congested Bay Area.

Another brother, Willie, who has since died, also visited me. His visit was a great surprise because we didn't often see him even though he lived in San Francisco. Somehow he found out about the surgery and brought me a lovely book of poetry. The poems were short, beautiful and soothing to read. Another time, he brought me a lovely ceramic bud vase with a rose in it. I knew these gifts represented a special effort on his part, and I'll always cherish that memory. I only wish I'd been more lucid to remember more of our conversations. He died of bone cancer in July of 2007, surrounded by his children, grandchildren, ex-wife and us, his sisters. After the funeral I gave the bud vase to his daughter Kathy. His last days were spent in her home with the most loving, tender care possible. *En pas descanses, hermano.* May you rest in peace, brother.

Maggie and Terri came to see Sylvia and me, along with other family members. One special visit was from a young couple, Angie and her husband John. They had firsthand knowledge of the problems of kidney failure. John had inherited a medical condition which caused his kidneys to fail at a young age. He'd undergone one transplant by this time and knew that another, and possibly a third, were also in store for him. His wife, Angie, daughter of long-time family friends, had witnessed John's problems and sustained him with much love and devotion. Since then, she's become a living kidney donor for her son, and the three currently are doing well. Not many could appreciate our situation as much as that married couple. Their unspoken awareness said much. I can still recall how affectionate they were during their visits.

On the fourth day in the hospital , the nurse offered me less than half a glass of wonderful, wet water! Dunking my cracked, peeling lips into the cup, I let them linger there for a few seconds before sipping. I felt my raw, parched lips swelling up like sponges.

The hovering nurse was vigilant. "Just a few small sips. No gulping. Just take it in gradually." In a lighter tone she added, "You'll have some breakfast this morning."

As much as I love eating, I was surprised at my lack of appetite. Hunger had not been as big an issue as drinking water. When the breakfast tray came in, I took a couple of spoonfuls of oatmeal, sipped some coffee and took one bite of toast. That was it. What I really wanted was the next half glass of water.

Since taking the first steps on the evening of the surgery, I'd been walking in my room several times during the day. On the third day, I found I could manage the path to the doorway and a short distance along the passageway to the nurses' desk. Fortunately, the catheter had been removed on day three without any discomfort. So I was also able to go back and forth to the bathroom by myself as needed—though not too speedily.

By this time, I felt strong enough to walk up the hallway to Sylvia's room. I wanted to look especially healthy for her. When I looked into the bathroom mirror, I didn't look any different to myself. I couldn't tell anything was missing, and I remember thinking how odd that seemed.

Luckily, Cynthia had insisted that I get a hair permanent before being hospitalized. She knew how I groused about my straight hair, so she gave me a gift certificate to the hair salon I went to. I had made the hair appointment on one of the weekends Sylvia came down from Stockton. While I was at the hair salon, Cynthia and Sylvia dropped by to check up on me. Cynthia made some funny comments about not being able to tolerate me with straight hair, and we all laughed. Sylvia jumped to my defense, but only after she'd finished laughing. They stayed a little while, then drove off to meet friends. My hairdresser, Tina, was impressed that my daughter had treated me to the perm. I explained how lucky I was to have a daughter who always managed to surprise me with just the right thing.

Having the luxury of not having to curl my hair, I simply brushed it into place. After putting on some lipstick, I ventured forth, pushing my trusty IV pole along with me. Peeking in to see if Sylvia was in, I stood proudly at the door and announced, "Your *nina* concedes victory. I owe you five."

Sylvia's face lit up, and I was pleasantly surprised. Her coloring had improved and there was less puffiness. She looked as if she were relaxing rather than convalescing. "*Mija*, you look good! How do you feel?" Her hair was in a tight, neat ponytail that made her look like a teenager. She had to be as pleased with the thinner face as I was—and with her recaptured spunk.

I tried walking as straight as possible and eased myself onto the side of her bed. It was higher than the chair and easier for me to manage.

"Oh, I feel good, *nina*. How about you?" The last part sounded like a plea. I tried to calm any distress she might be feeling.

"I'm coming along pretty good, they say. Just not as fast as I used to be, that's all. That's what I get for being older. Say, I saw you zipping along the hall yesterday. You were really jammin'." It took no effort to be cheerful.

Her lovely eyes were reflective. "Yes, well, you know it was easier on me than on you. I haven't been down to visit you so you could rest. But I keep asking the nurses at the desk about you. They say you're doing fine. Do you really feel fine, *nina?*"

"Of course I do. I'm pretty sore here and there and a bit slower. But I feel a little better and stronger each day. And they say my creatinine levels are getting better and better. Your doctor and another doctor named Roberts have checked me out and say that I'm recovering well. I'm afebrile, whatever that means. I'm getting what I need for pain, so everything's on track. What about you?"

If there was anyone who understood creatinine numbers, it was Sylvia. "My creatinine level is good, too, and my urine production is up to speed. Your kidney is doing a great job for me, *nina*. And, oh, it feels sooooo good."

If I could have, I'd have jumped for joy. "And no more dialysis. I'm so glad." I squeezed her hand. "See. Didn't I tell you He'd watch over us?" I gently tapped her hand as she nodded. "Now, you're not forgetting to have some Hershey Kisses, are you?"

"I put them out for the nurses, *nina*. I'm not that much of a chocolate eater."

"Oh, my poor kidney! Don't blame me if it starts getting withdrawal symptoms. Can't relate to not being fond of chocolate, *mija*, sorry."

The relief of seeing her doing so well was deeply heartwarming, but I was pooped. "Gotta go. This is the farthest I've walked, and I'm bushed."

As I slowly got up she said, "I'll come to see you before dinner, before company comes."

Sylvia's visitors were, of course, younger than mine—and livelier. They started streaming in about the time the rattling of dinner trays sounded, although Sylvia didn't have to eat hospital food. They brought in treats from places like Taco Bell, Burger King or McDonald's, accompanied by shakes, chips and all kinds of junk food. She wasn't a big eater, but she loved fast food, and her friends knew it. Some of them would even call before leaving their jobs to see what her taste buds felt like having that particular evening. Cynthia and Terri were among the greatest perpetrators. I can still see the three of them tossing down all those carbs while laughing about anything and everything. For those moments, they were carefree—good medicine in itself.

Sylvia was very much into enjoying the now of any moment, and exulting in it for all it was worth. Terri and Cynthia were perfect company. One of her best friends, Elisa, also visited and joined in the upbeat mood. It was an enormous relief after the weeks preceding surgery, not only for Sylvia, but for all those who loved her. We had our old Sylvia back, and weren't we thrilled!

As Sylvia's progress and stats showed improvement, my own mobility increased. We often visited and walked the hallways together. My walks were fewer and shorter, but she'd pop in daily with that springy, jaunty walk of hers and ask, "Feel like going for a walk, *nina?*"

"Sure," I'd say, whether I felt like it or not, wanting to demonstrate how my condition was rapidly improving. She still took naps, but the in-between times witnessed a more vibrant young woman, one eager to get back to normal routines. That eagerness filled me with an overwhelming sense of contentment. Any discomfort I was experiencing dissipated at seeing, listening to or thinking of her.

Many times the giver often benefits more than the recipient. That's certainly how I felt. The dread that, for some reason, my kidney might prove inadequate left me. So did the anxiety of failing Sylvia. Those rainy January days exuded a special sunshine within me, especially since I saw it mirrored in her face, too. One always appreciates faith when one's prayers are answered. At this stage, we were aglow with thanksgiving.

The tough part comes when one perceives that one's prayers haven't been answered. That struggle was still ahead.

15

The Great Care at UCSF

The learning experience from our surgery was profound, leaving me with a sense of wonder. For instance, I learned about the workings of my elimination system. Normally, who pays much attention to the act of urinating, its color, quantity and frequency? I know I sure didn't. And I'd say most people don't. Since the removal of the catheter, I was required to pee into a plastic container placed underneath the toilet lid in my bathroom. Immediately after voiding into it, I found myself analyzing what I had created. The amounts weren't as generous as normal, but I was greatly relieved to find no pain associated with urinating post surgery. The normal function of urinating is an important barometer of our health, and both the testing and post-operative periods emphasized that.

At regular intervals, nurses would collect the urine and pass it on to the lab. A constant reminder to drink plenty of water was the daily gospel, and I tried my best to comply. My creatinine levels were improving. The wound was clean, and I was moving easier, though still slower than normal.

Pain management occupied a lot of my attention in the days following surgery. I tried to evaluate how much it was lessening each day. Looking back, I realize that the idea of pain was stronger than the reality of it. I was so alert to preventing it, I probably gave it too much emphasis, especially the first two days after surgery. This is not to say the surgery was painless. There was some, but it was tolerable. When I thought pain might become unbearable, I asked for, and received, pain medication. In addition, I had access to the fabulous zapper that released its magic elixir. Having my zapper was a wonderful security blanket. Pressing the button became a reflex, especially before getting out of bed or up from a chair.

My main complaint was the swelling and discomfort throughout my abdominal area. It looked and felt as if I'd just delivered a nine-pound baby and retained the afterbirth. Also present was the same type of soreness and swelling in the stomach area, similar to postpartum. I hadn't expected to see my stomach puff out. My organs, intestines and nerve endings seemed traumatized at having been poked at, and they were letting me know it. Again, in looking back, the sensation was mostly discomfort, and it gradually diminished as each day passed. The actual incision wasn't bothersome. The doctors assured me that as the inflammation inside lessened, my stomach's size would return to normal. In the meantime, I was to drink plenty of water and walk about as much as possible—and drink plenty of water.

The post-operative phases I went through are ancient history when compared with today's. I mention them only because, at the time of my surgery, they were part of my personal experience. Today the body is not exposed to as much trauma. Microsurgery is used and the incision area is much smaller. Progress in transplanting organs has come a long way. Many of the symptoms and aches I felt simply are no longer part of the donor experience. It's a whole different procedure, with entirely different and better effects on the recuperation phase of the surgery. Less intrusive techniques translate into less pain, less trauma to the body and faster recuperation. If ever there was a time to be a living donor, it's now.

About three days after surgery, I heard the nurses say that the IV had to be repositioned or removed entirely, depending upon what the doctor advised. You can imagine my panic. The morphine drip, on which I felt so dependent, was about to be taken out. Having the IV reinserted during surgery had proven extremely satisfactory. It wasn't at all uncomfortable anymore and didn't bother me no matter how much I moved. The thought of repeating the first day's scenario of failed IV insertion attempts was unpleasant. I got quite disturbed. The day passed, however, without that happening.

About the fourth day, my nurse bounced into the room to take my vital readings and announced, "We're going to have to give you more potassium. Your levels are low. We'll do it through the IV." She wound the blood pressure band around my upper arm, then clamped a plastic clothespin-lookalike to my index finger to measure the oxygen in my blood. This was a new gadget for me, and I was amazed that this odd little tool could work merely by being attached to a finger. Apparently, high levels of oxygen in one's blood speed healing. Lack of oxygen inhibits healing. Oxygen level became an additional vital sign to be monitored. Blood pressure was great, pulse normal, oxygen level satisfactory. The nurse jotted down the numbers in the binder, rechecked what she'd entered, slammed the medical record shut, and inspected the IV needles.

"I'm going to get the potassium to put into the IV." She paused for a moment. "Just to let you know, sometimes there's a burning sensation. So let me know right away and I'll slow down the rate of intake, which should lessen the effect. Okay?" She patted my leg and departed.

True to her word, she returned, inserted the contents of a packet into the IV, and encouraged me to buzz for her if it became uncomfortable. About fifteen minutes later, I buzzed.

"It's really starting to burn. Did you put chili power in there?" I tried for humor as I hate sounding like a whiner.

She reached for the flow regulator on the IV stand and adjusted it. "There, I've slowed it up. That should make it better."

Wrong! The burning increased past the edge of tolerance, and for the first time, I felt I was losing it. My blood had turned to lava, and I expected to see it erupting any second. I pressed the buzzer again, and she reappeared almost immediately. I begged her to remove the IV.

"I'll take a shot of potassium, pills, anything, but get this out of me. I can't stand it!" It was all I could do to keep from screaming.

"I'll have to get the doctor's approval to do that."

"Get it, please. This is awful. They said I'd only need this IV for three or four days. It's been that already. I'm drinking and eating. Can't I take this stuff orally?"

My legs flexed up and down beneath the thin blanket as if by their movement, the pain in my hand and arm would go away. My free hand clutched the rail. She left, hopefully to get the doctor's approval to remove the IV.

An eternity of fifteen minutes elapsed before my nurse returned. She took my hand and gently withdrew the needles. The grimace on my face got me a compassionate, "There, there. It's out, the pain'll be gone in a little bit. The doctor says it's all right to give you the potassium orally." She seemed as relieved as I was. There is absolutely nothing as reassuring or comforting as a good nurse when one is hospitalized, and she was a good one.

I was afraid to say anything for fear of sobbing. The relief in my veins was only gradual. But I knew the source of the misery was gone, and the torment would eventually be gone. What a relief! Slowly, the realization that I was liberated from the IV connection sank in. Now I really felt I was on the road to recovery. With a sigh, I sank back into my pillow.

As it turned out, having won the battle of removing the IV didn't mean I was free from combat. An unsuspecting young resident doctor (or intern) appeared about an hour later to announce that he was going to have another IV put in. The poor creature could never have imagined the impact of his statement. His words went to the very depths of my soul.

"Oh, no, you don't! Dr. Melzer said I'd only need it for three or four days. This is the fourth day and you're NOT putting it back in. The nurse got permission to take it out, and it's staying out. You go check with her and see. I'm not letting anyone put in another one of those things unless Melzer absolutely insists on it. I don't know why I need it any more. I'll drink gallons of water if you want. I'm taking pain medication orally now, so why can't I take anything else you want me to swallow? No more IVs!" My words ricocheted off the walls.

The resident doctor stood rigid, hands on the bed railing, his eyes focused on something outside my window. He firmly restated, "You'll have to have another one."

Raising myself a bit higher than the already sitting-up position I was in, I clenched my teeth and softly, but quite emphatically, snarled, "If Melzer tells me I must, then I will. Otherwise, nobody's putting it back in."

He just kept standing there, then he relaxed a bit. "Oh, well, if Dr. Melzer said it was all right, then it's probably fine."

He nodded towards me and left. I've never felt so ferocious in my life, nor known as much relief once he left. It was pretty shameful of me, I suppose, but it's what happened. In retrospect, I think it was all the result of feeling vulnerable and powerless. Whatever the reason, at the time I had no regrets about fighting for what I felt were my rights. Still, I do feel I owe this poor young doctor an apology. If I knew his name, I would say I was sorry for my rude manner that day. Hopefully, in his career he has not encountered too many distressed patients ready to commit "physiciancide."

By the fifth day, I could promenade around our portion of the floor corridor twice in the morning and once in the afternoon and evening. The swelling around my stomach was going away, as was the bloated feeling. A lumbering gait remained. Every time I twisted or turned I was careful to do it slowly. But even that was getting easier. I must have looked like I was walking underwater, Jacques Cousteau style. I attempted no sudden movements, and the motto was, "Easy does it."

Anyone who's ever been hospitalized is aware that doctors and nurses are obsessed with bowel movements after surgery. It's absolutely imperative that one be achieved prior to dismissal. Every day, the first question upon entering the room is, "Have you had a BM yet?" I felt I was letting them down in some way until, finally, I was able to utter those magic words: "I had a BM!" I almost expected to hear applause and the adulation parents of toddlers bestow upon their potty-training offspring. I was surprised it wasn't announced over the PA system.

Okay, so I'm being facetious. Attention to all these functions acknowledges the expertise, skill and commitment that we are privileged to receive from our doctors, nurses, technicians and health administrators. Frankly, I'm awed by it. I can't think of any other word to use, although thankful comes to mind. I remember many things that comforted me during those days in the hospital, from the caring tone of a voice, to the repeated encouragement and assurances, to the small considerate gestures and spontaneous outpouring of caring that made the whole experience miraculously successful.

Without a doubt, the staff and facility at UCSF are at the cutting edge of science and new technology aimed at improving the human condition. The knowledge that I was in the best possible medical facility in our area for the type of surgery Sylvia and I had had instilled great trust. It never faltered. Receiving sustained medical attention twenty-four hours a day is an extraordinary experience. I'd heard Sylvia rave about her doctors. When I left, I completely understood and shared her feelings for them, and for every person involved in our pre-op, post-op and follow-up care.

16

Joint Recuperation

Six days after surgery, I left the hospital. In reviewing my medical files years later, Dr. Melzer's notes read: "Patient was seen and examined, and the case was discussed with the transplant team. Patient is being discharged today following donor nephrectomy. Wound is healing well. She is afebrile and has normal bowel function. She will be followed in the transplant clinic." I've since learned that afebrile means "not marked by fever."

So, on January 16th, I was discharged. Sylvia remained because she needed a few additional days for regulation of her medications and further monitoring of creatinine levels. Her doctors also needed to make sure that the new kidney continued to behave properly. It was gratifying to know that it had been functioning admirably from the start. The doctors told me that it wasn't uncommon for transplanted kidneys to wait days before beginning to function. Mine had kicked in within minutes of being placed inside Sylvia. I was proud of my kidney, but the joy of seeing her regaining her health was the most rewarding feeling imaginable.

On the morning before I left, I stopped by Sylvia's room. She was in great spirits and moving about with more agility than I. Ah, youth.

"I can't wait to get to the townhouse, too, *nina*. Got to give the princess a hard time."

"Three more days and you'll get that chance, *mija*. In the meantime, be good. Don't forget to eat your veggies and a Hershey Kiss every night.

Remember, we've got to be on a healthy diet when you get out, you know." I leaned over to kiss her forehead. "See you soon. I'll call you after I get home."

Joe had taken time off work to pick me up and was also in Sylvia's room. They kidded around for a while, as usual. After giving her a loving peck and hug, we were off. As Joe and I walked down the hallway arm in arm, we passed the bustling nurses' station. This gave me an opportunity to thank them again for their excellent care. I certainly found out the importance of good nursing and will never forget it. I left my phone number at the nurses' desk and told them if I could be of any help to a nervous prospective donor, I'd be happy to talk with him or her. They seemed glad for the offer and wished me well.

As we continued on our way out, it occurred to me that I'd been one of only two living donors on the floor during the past week. A husband and wife had been there briefly, but I didn't know anything else about their situation. Other than that, the few other patients on our floor were recipients of deceased persons' organs or were kidney patients interned to be stabilized with new medication or revised dosages of their present meds. This lack of live donors struck me as odd, especially since I knew how many people were on the organ waiting lists. I remember thinking, "If only they knew how easy it was." Since I was so excited about going home, I didn't give the matter more thought until years later.

What an experience! I was exhilarated by the success of the surgery and at being released. Next to giving birth, it's the closest I've felt to nurturing life. It was such a high! Everything that had preceded surgery had been worthwhile. The strain of the prolonged testing, the mini-bouts of anxiety, the aftermath of surgery, and even the IV ordeal faded away.

And in a few days Sylvia would also be leaving the hospital. There was no way I could imagine the depth of her feelings. No more dialysis, no more tackle box full of meds, no more lethargy. Would it be like being reborn? Only someone who'd walked in her shoes could relate to being healthy again. I hoped she'd be as lightheaded with joy as I felt now.

As Joe drove home, I stole a side glance at him. Like most mothers, my eyes never tire of the sight of my children. Even when they were little, I could hardly take my eyes off of them for fear I'd miss some incredible new facial expression, gesture or brilliant act. Now that they were adults, I sneaked looks at them as inconspicuously as possible. I could tell that Joe was driving with extra care. He looked serious, but happy.

Everyone looked happy that day. The trees along Sunset Drive were glossy from previous rains, and the cool air held a crispness. As we turned the bend in Daly City onto Interstate 280, the bay came into view —another sight I can't get my fill of. Before I knew it, we'd reached the driveway of the townhouse. The garage door opened by remote, and Joe slowed to a gentle stop.

"Wait for me to open the door, Mom. Let's take our time." Joe eased the car partway into the garage so that I'd have plenty of room to walk in front of it.

The townhouse felt so welcoming. From the foyer I slowly climbed upstairs and found that Cynthia had placed all the plants, cards and flowers from well-wishers on the dining room table. The scent was lovely, as was the view I'd missed so much. The world looked newly washed, and the muted blues of the bay were speckled with whitecaps. A few clouds traveled over the water, their shadows darkening the bay. Every day at these windows seems to create a new panorama of melding sky, water and earth. I had missed the ever-changing scenery. I sighed with contentment.

Joe returned from depositing my overnight bag in the bedroom. "Mom, let's go downstairs and get you settled in. Want something to drink?"

Joe's arm supported me to the lower floor. Still in my robe, I eased onto the bed while he propped a couple of pillows behind me. The bed tray from Christmas was on one side of the bed with the paper folded neatly on top of it. After making sure that a water pitcher and glass were on the nightstand, he settled on the bed. He opened up the sports section for a few moments before laying it back down. "Mom, I'm glad it's over."

"Yep, me too, *mijo*. And didn't it turn out good?"

He simply nodded. For an instant, I wanted to apologize for putting him through the worry of the surgery. But I didn't regret it, so how could I express regret?

I smiled at him. "Thanks for bringing me home, *mijo*. I know how busy you are at work. Thank your boss for me, too, okay?"

"Mom, you know I'm glad to do it." Then a bit more seriously, he added, "Besides, Cindy would've killed me if I hadn't."

We both laughed. He was probably right. He must have asked me if I needed anything else half a dozen times. Finally, I told him to scoot. "Cynthia will be home in a couple of hours. I'll be fine." I opened my arms for an embrace.

He leaned over and planted a kiss on my cheek. "I'll call you later tonight. Be good, Mom."

Once I heard the garage door close, I nestled back and fell asleep.

Sylvia was released a few days later and, as planned, came to the townhouse to recuperate. Her face was even thinner than earlier in the week when I'd left the hospital. The smile was back in her eyes, and her body was returning to its former shape. She shared Cynthia's upper bedroom. We quickly settled into a comfortable routine. Cynthia made sure we had fresh water, some fruit and the paper each morning before she left for work. Prior to being hospitalized, I'd filled the pantry and freezer with easy, ready-to-eat foods that Sylvia and I fixed ourselves. It wasn't difficult to do minor chores like light cooking and washing dishes. After all, we weren't incapacitated, just slow. I was still the slower of the two, though gradually gaining ground.

Sylvia and I concentrated on regaining our strength. Actually, the torpid pace suited us both. We awoke at our leisure, ate and drank with nutrition in mind, napped, read, watched TV and even took two daily walks. By this time it was the end of January. Day after day it rained. Nevertheless, our doctors had adamantly instructed us to walk at least twenty minutes twice a day, and we complied in spite of the weather. At mid-morning, we slipped on our tennis shoes, put raincoats on over our bathrobes or sweats, grabbed an umbrella and strolled around our short street for twenty minutes. I felt comical in my purple paisley-patterned robe, maroon sweats, lavender raincoat and Reeboks. Sylvia usually wore sweats and tennis shoes, but no raincoat. Actually, it was rather freeing to disregard color coordination or fashion.

Carrying our umbrellas, we strode past the mailboxes, the soggy patches of lawns and the swaying, perpetually-shedding eucalyptus trees. From one end of the complex's mini-street to the other, we made our way along until it was time to turn around. Sylvia would fling her umbrella aside, close her eyes, lift her head skyward, and offer her face to the rain.

"Oh, *nina*, I love the rain on my face! Walking in the rain is soooo cool." Her tiny nose scrunched with delight. "It feels so soft." She shook her head and her chestnut tresses, darkened by moisture, whipped from side to side.

The first time she did this, I chided, "*Mija*, you're getting soaked." In truth, I got as much pleasure from her uplifted face as she did. For Sylvia, these were lovely moments free of pain, a future free of dialysis machines and full of hope. She was in what Don calls "gleemania." It showed in her outstretched hands cupped to receive the raindrops, and in her light step as she sprang forward. It was like walking with a leprechaun, a mischievous imp that had rediscovered life and seized it as if it were the proverbial pot of gold. To this day, that is one of my favorite mental images of her.

For two weeks, we walked twice a day for twenty minutes, and each day the number of round-trips around the tiny street increased from two to three to four. Our pace was definitely improving. I yearned to go up the hill to Crystal Springs Trail along the San Andreas Fault on Skyline Drive, where I had enjoyed walking before the surgery. The trail is three miles round-trip, an ideal length for moderate exercise. As soon as I could drive, I promised myself I'd revisit the rolling path along the reservoir. Maybe I'd even see some mule deer grazing behind the protection of the barbed-wired fencing separating the watershed from the path.

Just as I craved getting back to my usual routine, Sylvia desired the same. She missed her dog, Freeway, and longed to wake up in her own bed. She looked forward to resuming a healthy lifestyle, even sharing in the household chores. There was much she looked forward to doing— and not doing.

"It's going to be great not having to go to dialysis, *nina*. And I can hardly wait to get back to work." She often talked about the Girl Scouts of America's office in Stockton and of the friends she'd made there and her supervisor. "They're so nice to me. And we have lots of fun while still getting our work done." From the way she talked, it was obvious she took a lot of pride in her job. What struck me was the eagerness in her voice. It had returned.

After our late morning constitutional, we usually watched some television in the den before our naps. Afterwards, I sat on the sofa with a TV tray propped in front of me. It spilled over with cards that needed acknowledging, along with some personal stationery and thank-you cards. Each day we wrote a few notes thanking people for whatever they'd sent or for their visits or phone calls. All the while, we chatted. Our conversations were easy, spontaneous and filled with humor.

"Stop, *mija*. You're making my insides jiggle." I found myself repeating this phrase a lot.

We bounced thoughts off each other, and the similarity in our thinking and opinions was evident—just as Maggie had so often said. If I became indignant over a news report or television program we happened to be watching, she'd continue my thought to the next level. "Not only that, but…" she would say, carrying the line of reasoning to the same conclusion I might have expressed. And when we saw or heard something that struck our funny bones, we convulsed in laughter. The quiet intervals in between were enjoyable, easy and comfortable.

Since her arrival from the hospital, whenever we spoke I couldn't take my eyes off her thinning face. It was beginning to match the graduation picture on the shelf in the den. The lilt in her voice toned her conversations as before. It was music to my ears. She was as funny as ever and giggling often. There's a saying in Spanish, *"Me llena el ojo,"* meaning, "she fills my eyes." It implies that one can see nothing else. That's the spell Sylvia had me under during our convalescence.

One day, while we were sitting on the sofa resting from our midday walk, she suddenly threw her arms around me and blurted out, "Oh, *nina*, I feel soooo good!" She started to cry. Sylvia rarely cried. Aside from my last birthday, the last time I'd seen her shed tears was when Mando had died years earlier. But this was a happy cry. I hugged her back. A profound warmth flowed between us.

"Ay, *nina*." She grabbed a tissue. "Whew! I don't know where that came from." Taking a few deep breaths, she said, "I think I'll take my nap now. Got to rest before the brat gets home."

There was no way of knowing how burdensome Sylvia's fears must have been prior to surgery, as she wasn't one to share her anxieties. Her worries for her health must have been incredible. Yet, as I watched her bounce up the stairs, remembering that day when she couldn't keep up with Terri and Cynthia, I knew all those fears were gone. Had today been the day when she'd truly felt a full recovery was hers? Was that what had brought on the sudden burst of tears? If so, letting me share in her epiphany was another precious gift from Sylvia. I don't think she ever suspected how much she enriched my life.

The renewed lightness in Sylvia's manner reminded me of how brave she'd been in the preceding months. The ravages of kidney failure are not easy to bear. She had endured them with immense courage and without complaint. How I admired her for it. Not only her, but Maggie, Terri and Gil also had been strong. The whole clan was pleased that Sylvia's ordeal had been resolved and she and her family could resume a normal life. I could hardly wait for them to see how vibrant she was again. For now, it felt special that Sylvia, Cynthia and I shared our convalescence privately. In a short while, everyone would share in the return of our Sylvia's health. Since our return from the hospital, the family had regularly called to ask about her progress. But when they could see it for themselves, I knew they'd be thrilled.

The princess had once again reverted to the brat. Sylvia and Terri were as close as sisters to Cynthia, and she loved them with a devotion never mentioned but continuously demonstrated. It was her bedroom that Terri and Sylvia shared whenever they drove down from Stockton. Behind those doors existed confidential headquarters, where feelings were shared, family gossip or "remembering" took place, plans were made and dreams were revealed. Lord knows what else was hashed out.

It was times like these when an occasional word in Spanish hit my ears. Of the three, Terri was the one who spoke Spanish the most. Of all the cousins, Cynthia spoke it the least. Normally our children spoke English exclusively unless in the presence of their grandparents. When I heard the girls use Spanish, I knew they were joking about something or using an expression that sounded funnier in Spanish than in English. There are some words that just sound more amusing in Spanish—or meaner.

Sylvia was a chronic snorer, and Cynthia teased her about it, but she cherished Sylvia's presence. They also indulged in verbal combat in the traditional Zertuche manner. They were keenly observant of weak spots in each other, which were quickly identified and exploited to their fullest. Honing their arguing skills on each other was a sport they enjoyed. Terri, the third part of the triangle, was a respected participant in this magic confab. In fact, when she was around, she was the combatant whose talent spurred the other two to keep in practice. The three occupied a special realm that only they understood. It was a cultivated, treasured bond exclusive of all others.

The brat was an attentive nurse. She didn't baby us. But she did make sure we had what we needed while checking that we didn't get too rambunctious. For the most part, we did things for ourselves—fixing light meals and tidying up. Such activity must have been beneficial, because by our second week home from the hospital, we were noticeably stronger. The tenderness inside my abdomen disappeared. A couple of weeks into recuperating, all I needed was an occasional Tylenol during the day and sometimes at night.

Surprisingly, the incision didn't bother me. Once the bandage was removed, I applied liquid Vitamin E to it to reduce the keloid (the lumpy, white scarring) effect in healing. A nurse at UCSF had suggested this ointment to minimize scarring. I continued applying the sticky oil for several months. As a result, the scar is hardly visible. It wasn't so much that I worried what the scar would look like. I've never had a bikini-type body. I just didn't want to feel a bulgy line along my side. Luckily, the Vitamin E worked.

I never saw Sylvia's scars. She'd told me sometime prior to our surgery that the surgeons didn't remove her original kidneys because they'd atrophied in place and didn't need to be taken out. When they transplanted both Terri's and my kidney, they placed them just under the skin in the front abdominal area. Sylvia said this frontal position facilitated access to the kidney in case her doctors needed to do a biopsy. It made sense to me. I didn't even ask if they'd removed Terri's failed kidney when putting in mine. If Sylvia didn't offer the information, I didn't want to pry it out of her.

I never showed her my scar because I sensed Sylvia's reluctance to look at anything which might have caused me pain. Neither of us had a curiosity about each other's incisions. I remember mentioning that I was using Vitamin E on the incision and told her it was in the medicine cabinet if she wanted it. All she said was, "Okay, *nina*. If I remember." Whether she ever did use it, I don't know.

This hesitancy to ask personal questions may seem odd in view of our close relationship. But part of that relationship included a respect for privacy. We both had a sense of what our personal boundaries were and never crossed over them. We enjoyed the other side too much. Ironically, I wouldn't have given the matter a second thought if she'd asked to see my incision. Maybe she just didn't feel comfortable asking. Another reason might have been modesty. Modesty was definitely a component in our daughters' lives. I'm sure with their peers, they were more relaxed about private matters or dressing and undressing in front of each other. This was especially true when we were all camping and the girls shared a tent. If that comfort level didn't extend to my generation, it didn't matter to me. I accepted it without the need for explanations.

About two weeks after being released from UCSF, Sylvia and I had follow-up visits at the hospital's transplant clinic. Cynthia drove us in for the first appointment. By the time of our second one two weeks after that, I drove myself and Sylvia in. We both checked out with high marks. Sylvia's progress surpassed expectations. Her creatinine levels were good, which meant that the kidney was doing its job. Each day saw increased energy levels. Her color was fabulous, the puffiness was almost gone, and the impish gleam in her eyes got brighter.

Seeing Sylvia rise to such healthy levels was such a high for me. It really brought home the feeling that the giver often receives more than the recipient. I almost felt guilty about the emotional gratification. Mostly, I was immensely thankful. Our prayers had been answered to the fullest.

My stats were just as good. The swelling about my stomach was notably reduced, and the wound had closed up and was scarring nicely. My creatinine levels were perfect.

Three weeks later, it was time for Sylvia to return to Stockton. Maggie and Terri had been burning up the telephone wires between their place and San Bruno. They were naturally eager to have her back. Terri had made it down to visit a couple of times while we were recuperating, but that was no substitute for Sylvia's daily presence at home. Sylvia, too, looked forward to going home to her dog and resuming a normal routine. The healthier she became, the more she chomped at the bit to go home.

Once the doctors advised her that she didn't have to go in for check-ups as often, she made plans to leave us. Cynthia teased Terri that the person Sylvia really missed was the dog. I certainly had conflicting feelings about her departure. I knew I'd miss her company, yet was mindful of how much she was looking forward to restarting her life.

As it turned out, the first week of February marked the end of our private odyssey. The days of singing and frolicking in the rain were over. This whole experience, from early November to February, remains one of the most treasured events of my life—most especially our joint convalescence. So many of those days remain sharp in my mind—the conversations, the reminiscences and the laughter. It's a lot to be thankful for.

On a non-gloomy, rainy February day, Sylvia and I stood arm in arm in the living room while Cynthia snapped our photo. As I look at that picture now, I ignore the slight chubbiness in Sylvia's cheeks and the hint of a moustache—effects of pre-surgery medications. Before long the traces left over from her pre-surgery days would disappear. That wonderful departure is seared into my mind, heart and soul. It signaled the success we'd prayed for and the promise of a healthier life for Sylvia. This was her new life—her healthy new life—and I was exuberant for her future. At least, that's what we all thought at the time.

"Don't be sad, *nina*. I'll be back the night before my next appointment. We'll see each other a lot over the next few weeks."

"Of course I'm not sad, *mija*. I'm just thinking, now that you're going, it means I'll have to return to work soon myself. Plus, I won't have anyone around to agree with me anymore." I threw Cynthia a meaningful glance.

Sylvia giggled. "You better be nice to my *nina*, brat," she threatened. "Or I'll sic Terri on you."

"Oh, and that's supposed to scare me? I don't think so," Cynthia said. "Besides, Mom needs a little conflict in her life, and I'm it. Somebody's got to do it."

Sylvia was so excited about going home that she didn't want to wait for the weekend, when either Cynthia could drive her or Terri could come down to pick her up. Instead, she and Terri had agreed that Sylvia would return by train and arrive in Stockton about the time Terri got off work.

"I've never ridden a train before, and it'll be fun to give it a whirl," Sylvia said, alive with enthusiasm.

"You're sure you'll be okay? You've got plenty of meds and…"

Cynthia broke in. "Mom, she'll be okay. Don't worry."

"Right, *nina*. Terri's picking me up at the station. I've timed it so I'll get there by four-thirty, which gives her plenty of time to get there after work. She's got the schedule and knows what train I'm taking. We're all set."

"Well, say hi to your mom for me and to Terri. And if you want, give Freeway a hug, too." A quick squeeze and she was off.

Cynthia drove her to the train station in San Francisco. The minute Sylvia walked out the front door, the house felt different. At the same time, I couldn't have been happier that her new life had just begun. But it reminded me of when my son Joe moved out. At twenty-four years old, it was time for him to be on his own. While I embraced his being prepared to strike out on his own, I missed him. That's what I felt when Sylvia left for Stockton. Everything pointed to its desirability, but there was a tinge of selfishness that yearned for her presence.

Sylvia's departure forced me to examine my own schedule. Being well on my way to normalcy meant that I had to think about returning to work. John was beginning to call about office matters. "Bel, where's the file on the truck terminal? Did they ever respond to our request for an update on the soil remediation?" Or, "When do we pay the Hana employees?"

Actually, I think he enjoyed any excuse to check up on me. He'd been worried about the outcome of the surgery and was probably greatly relieved to know that I'd be able to go back to work at the end of the allotted six weeks' time just as healthy as ever.

On my last day of work prior to surgery, I'd made John promise not to visit me in the hospital, as I knew his legs bothered him a great deal. Hospital hallways were much too long for his aching limbs. In addition, walking from the parking lot to the hospital through the vast labyrinth of the medical center would also have been an ordeal for him. He chose instead frequent telephone calls.

How many times have we told ourselves not to take one another for granted? To appreciate family and friends? To say "I love you" often? If only I would have practiced that precious tenet with my boss and friend before he died. The guilt I feel for never having told him how important he was to me or how much his welfare mattered haunts me. It simply never occurred to me that he would die later that spring. John was the epitome of integrity, a worthy steward of the responsibilities entrusted to him and an astute financial manager. His example serves me well to this day, and it was my good fortune to have had him influence my life in such a meaningful manner.

Did I mention his sense of humor? John was half Irish, half German, and an all-around fan of a funny story. He liked a good laugh, good company, and a strong drink when not working. He and the late Don Sherwood, a famous San Francisco disc jockey, were fishing buddies. John was also Sherwood's accountant and executor. Anyone familiar with Don Sherwood's career is aware of how hysterically funny and outrageous he was during his time on KSFO radio in San Francisco. He had radio's early morning commute market sewn up tight in the Bay Area through the fifties and sixties.

As a Highway 101 commuter, I can attest to the messy traffic that was the norm on that corridor leading into the city. I think every car had their radio tuned in to KSFO. It wasn't uncommon for commuters to hear one of Don's funny or outrageous remarks and burst out laughing while trying to maneuver the clogged freeway or while stuck in a traffic jam. With a turn of our heads, we could see that fellow drivers were also enjoying the same joke or comment. His popularity as a DJ remains unmatched in the Bay Area.

Don Sherwood was one of a kind, as was John. That they enjoyed each other's company attests to John's sense of humor and Don's good judgment. By the time John and I had been thrust together by the McAllister Trust, Don had died. John sometimes spoke of their fishing trips, and it was obvious they were a treasured part of his past. They both loved deep-sea fishing along the California and Mexican coasts from the San Francisco Bay to Baja California. Both had fishing boats. When Sherwood died, John really missed his fishing buddy. I don't think he ever enjoyed his boat or fishing as much after that.

At about five weeks after surgery, I was beginning to wish for additional time at home. That was a sure sign of getting my health back. Apart from maternity leave and a short period when the kids were toddlers, and another respite in the mid-eighties, I'd been a working mom with only two weeks off per year plus eight holidays. During my convalescence I enjoyed the new experience of waking up at a leisurely pace and not having to bathe and dress in a mad rush while dreading the morning commute. Reading the paper while the news was still fresh was another perk I relished. This latest routine was really beginning to agree with me. I began missing it before actually going back to work. But that reality couldn't be postponed much longer.

I checked in with Sylvia a few times after she left and was thrilled at how quickly she'd gotten back into her working routine. She loved her job as administrative assistant with the Girl Scouts of America, as she had often told me while we were convalescing. She especially appreciated how understanding they had been when she missed work. Being able to return to her job meant more to Sylvia than I realized at the time. Hearing her enthusiasm about it was heartening.

"It's great being back, *nina.*" She giggled when telling me that she felt so good, they were piling on the work. "Ay, *nina*, I'm really busy." If words could smile, these were. This really convinced me that Sylvia's renewed healthy status had retriggered her life. Now that she was back in the saddle, I called less frequently. But I got updates on Sylvia from Cynthia, who regularly spoke with Terri and reported back to me. It seemed things were truly back to normal.

Too quickly, the six weeks of recovery were up, and the time for me to report back to the office arrived on schedule in mid-February. The first week back, I put in approximately four hours per day, after which I was eager to leave for my afternoon nap. The second week's four-hour stint became easier, so I started working five hours. Within three weeks I was back to the normal forty-hour work week as if I'd never been gone. I resumed my lunchtime walks around Richardson's Bay. By March tenth, the two-month anniversary of our surgery, I was pretty much back to normal. A month later, my old habit of taking after-work walks along the Crystal Springs Skyline Trail resumed once the rains quit.

Gradually, my previous energy levels came back, my stomach deflated, the tenderness disappeared, and except for rubbing Vitamin E onto the scar, there were no residual effects from surgery. The remaining kidney functioned well and was maintaining my body's filtering system at top efficiency. The nerve endings were happy again, and my life became a mirror of what it had been three months earlier. By looking at me and seeing me in action, no one would have guessed that I'd ever had major surgery, much less a nephrectomy. Frankly, even to this day, I forget I only have one kidney. Except for one important occasion. Any time I get a new prescription, I ask the doctor if it will affect my kidney. That's the only time I make an issue of having one kidney. Fortunately, I don't have to take much medication. That one can give up an organ without detriment to oneself has to be one of nature's most amazing marvels. It certainly remains a source of wonderment to me.

With both Sylvia and I in our familiar daily routines, life became wonderfully normal—and more appreciated. It was a time of great thanksgiving for all our family. If only it could have lasted.

17

False Alarm

Organ rejection is a common concern with any transplant patient, and the doctors are careful to prepare both recipient and donor for that possibility. From the very beginning of the process I was aware that rejection by the organ recipient could occur. Even though Sylvia had been able to accept my kidney and it had functioned well from the onset, the potential still existed. For this reason, she was routinely scheduled for check-ups and testing. The immediate success of the surgery and the positive results experienced afterwards lulled us into complacency—until April of the same year, when we were rudely shaken up.

Sylvia was readmitted to UCSF Medical Center the following April because she was experiencing what might have been signs of rejection. Her creatinine levels had inexplicably risen. The Stockton Kaiser doctors suspected that a new liver transplant medication that was being tried on kidney transplant patients was the culprit. They immediately referred her to UCSF. As previously mentioned, too much creatinine in our system means that the kidney is not doing a proper job of filtering the body's waste. Most of us have creatinine levels hovering between one and two points, which is the norm. Hers were up past six points. Something was wrong, and she needed immediate re-evaluation at UCSF. They promptly took a biopsy of her (my "ex") kidney.

Our hearts sank at the possibility Sylvia was experiencing rejection. Our emotions had gone from euphoria back to gloom. Seeing her back in the hospital after what had been a successful transplant operation was terrifying. When we visited her, we tried to hide our fears. Though she didn't express them, similar thoughts must have preoccupied her even more. Typically, she appeared positive. Still, she was puzzled. "I don't think I did anything different. All of a sudden, I just didn't feel good. Ay, *nina*. I wish they'd hurry up with the results of the biopsy."

We concentrated on being positive and tried to boost her spirits with encouraging words. Fortunately, within a very short time they zeroed in on the problem. It was as the Stockton Kaiser clinic had suspected. It turned out that the solution lay in simply adjusting her medications. The analyses had taken a few days, and once the doctors were assured that the modification in dosage had kicked in properly, Sylvia was discharged. Whew!

Once Sylvia's condition had been diagnosed and treated that April, she left the hospital within a few days and returned to us in San Bruno. We all breathed easier, retreating into the comfortable cocoon of thinking all was well again.

When the scare had first surfaced, Cynthia was the one who informed me that Sylvia needed to return to UCSF. Terri had called her from Stockton to ask her to meet her and Sylvia at McDonald's in Tracy, a small town located on the junction close to Interstate 5. From there, Cynthia brought Sylvia to the hospital, saving Terri a trip all the way into the city. It was important for Terri not to miss work, so it became routine for her to call Cynthia with a brief "Meet me in Tracy" message. There was no elaboration, just a quick hang-up. Cynthia took it from there and met her cousins at McDonald's. Cynthia would then call me, and I knew to meet them at UCSF. It was a familiar routine. Now that we knew it'd been a false alarm, we were relieved she was back on track. That time she only stayed with us for a couple of days, just enough time to report back to the clinic for final monitoring before being allowed to return home to Stockton.

Once we knew things were under control, it became an enjoyable visit, and we resumed our chummy existence. The moment Sylvia received the green light from the transplant clinic, she left. She hated being away from her job, which was typical of her.

"*Nina*, I've already missed so much work, and they've been so good about it. I hate taking more time off." She ran her hand through her hair, reminding me of her dad.

"Well, I think they know you're not taking advantage of them, *mija*. After all, it's not like you're faking."

I knew exactly how she felt. I'd feel the same way in her shoes. Fortunately, she was able to go back with only one week's absence. Once our initial alarm was calmed by the easy resolution of med adjustment, the episode took on the aspect of a normal occurrence with this type of surgery. It was one that had been predicted, awaited, endured and corrected. It was simply a blip on the path to recovery. On the whole, my ex-kidney continued to respond favorably to the adjustments in her medications. Once again, I found myself sending her back home with encouraging words.

A couple of weeks after this incident, I called her at work and she sounded bright, bubbly and back in the swing of things. Such chats made my heart smile, easing any anxiety that occasionally surfaced. I so wanted my kidney to be perfect for her that any hint that it might malfunction bothered me. The slightest glitch in its condition seemed like a personal affront. Happily, her voice on the telephone was an accurate barometer for me. From it, I could tell that she was feeling well.

Cynthia's frequent conversations in the following weeks, mostly with Terri, gave me bits of information about Sylvia's progress. Lots of their chatter dealt with day-to-day occurrences and topics that young women discuss, not all of which are shared with parents. Basically, I was interested in how Sylvia was feeling, and Cynthia kept me posted on that. My live-in reporter did such a good job, I didn't have many person-to-person exchanges with Sylvia following her April visit.

Sometime in early May, Cynthia relayed that Sylvia wasn't feeling well and had gone to the doctor in Stockton. Transplant patients must take immunosuppressants for the remainder of their lives. Cyclosporine, tacrolimus, and sirolimus are three that are used. In addition, Prednisone

185

may also be prescribed. Additional medications such as mycopheolate, mofetil or azathioprine are sometimes used, at least during the time of Sylvia's second transplant. These all serve to guard against organ rejection by the recipient's immune system of what it perceives to be a foreign object in the body. Immunosuppressants affect the body in different ways. Every individual reacts in his or her own way.

Whatever the reason, Sylvia's health started to decline. The first Friday in May, Terri called Cynthia in tears, saying that she was on her way to UCSF with her sister. The doctors in Stockton were concerned about Sylvia's rising creatinine levels and insisted she return to the clinic for evaluation. Terri would drop Sylvia off at UCSF and then come to our place for the night.

When I heard the news, my heart immediately went out to Terri, who once again was deeply affected by her sister's health problems. She voiced no complaints, but it must have exacted heavy mental and spiritual effort to sustain that level of care and support to Sylvia. For my *comadre* Maggie, too, it couldn't have been easy to witness both daughters under the same umbrella of stress.

I knew from my conversations with Sylvia that she was bothered by the fact that her illness caused them so much worry. I tried to assure her no one felt burdened by her needs and that we realized they were not of her making. Still, it was a sentiment Sylvia often expressed to me. Clearly, none of us ever signaled any frustration or annoyance with Sylvia's circumstance. Our response was to help her get her health restored as quickly as possible. All our energies were expended to that end. No one showed impatience or indulged in reproaches. No one except Sylvia.

This time, I heard the news about Terri's trip to UCSF while I was at work. Cynthia called me just to let me know she was going to the hospital directly after work. Don and I had plans to meet for dinner, and I offered to cancel them.

"Mom, there's nothing you can do. According to Terri, Sylvia's really sleepy, not feeling good and probably not up to seeing anyone. I'm going up to keep Terri company and get her to come back with me at a decent hour. We'll probably grab a bite on the way home, so why don't you go ahead with your plans and we'll talk in the morning?"

Sometimes she sounded wise beyond her years. I agreed, but said that I'd be home extra early.

The next morning, which was a Saturday, the three of us were sitting in Cynthia's room on her bed, mugs of coffee in our hands. Terri, noticeably strained by Sylvia's latest condition, started talking, wiping away the falling tears as she spoke.

"She's just so sleepy. She started getting really tired again a couple of days ago." Terri took a sip of coffee as I shoved the box of tissues closer to her. "She did seem better, *tia*, when we left her room last night. They think it might just be another med adjustment problem, but they're going to take a biopsy of the kidney just to be sure." I wondered if she had said that to bolster my spirits or if it were really true.

With a near-laugh between sobs, Terri continued, "She made me promise to bring her a glazed donut this morning." Cynthia and I chuckled at that.

"Yep. You know she's better if her cravings kick in," Cynthia said.

"When do you have to be home, Terri? How about work?" I asked.

"I'm going to find out what's going on with her first, *tia*," she said. "Hopefully, by Monday I can get back, 'cause I've used up all my sick leave and I don't have any vacation time accumulated yet."

Terri had started a new job with a local medical clinic in Stockton, which was a step up from her previous employment. I knew she didn't want to be gone any more than necessary. Still, her first priority remained Sylvia.

Trying to be supportive, I said, "You know we can handle it from here if we need to, *mija*."

She nodded. We cut our talk short so that Cynthia and Terri could get ready. They wanted to pick up the donut and get to the hospital and be with Sylvia as soon as possible. I did a few chores at home, then followed them up early in the afternoon. The tension this was causing Terri worried me. When I arrived at the hospital, I found Sylvia cheerful, but weakened by an obvious lack of energy.

"Hi, *nina*. Oh, you shouldn't have come. It's not that important. I'll be okay. Some silly dosage mix-up, probably, that'll…" A big yawn interrupted her in mid-sentence "…get straightened out tomorrow." An uneaten donut lay on her tray.

She looked pale and sleepy. A weak smile formed and she leaned back on her pillows, one arm stretched over her head. With the hint of a twinkle in her eye, she tattled on her cousin. "*Nina*, scold Cindy. She's being mean to me. She says that Ginger" (our recently deceased family dog) "was smarter than Freeway will ever be."

"Sorry, *mija*, can't argue with that. But if you want, I'll give her a smack, anyway." I playfully slapped Cynthia's wrist.

"Hey! It's true." Her voice was saucy, but not the dark brown eyes that reflected her concern for Sylvia.

We sat around making small talk. When Sylvia nodded off, we exchanged worried glances. Terri and Cynthia took a break to go down to the cafeteria for a late lunch. I plopped down in the hospital chair, trying to shake off the heaviness in my heart. I concluded that Monday would define whatever was wrong. For now I squelched other possibilities, denying any might exist. The girls returned and, in hushed voices, we discussed our plans.

"Mom's on her way down," Terri said. "She should be here in a couple of hours."

"She can stay with us, you know that, *mija*," I said.

"Oh, thank you, *tia*. But I think she's staying with my *tia* Chu" (Maggie's sister). "I might go with her, I don't know yet."

"Whatever you decide is fine," I said.

Terri leaned back in her chair, eyes closed. I wondered if she was truly resting or going over different scenarios in her mind. Cynthia was also quiet. During the silence the girls occasionally rallied to exchange a barb, as if allowing too much time to lapse between cutting remarks would make them rusty. Sylvia woke up, smiled and straightened up.

"Did I doze off again? Brat, see what's on TV."

Cynthia surfed the limited television channels, and they argued about which program to watch. A few minutes into the program, Sylvia drifted off again.

During one of Sylvia's naps, Terri and I walked out into the hallway. I could see that these emergency forays into UCSF were taking their toll on her. Besides the emotional anxiety of repeatedly seeing her sister ill and being unsure of how serious the cause or causes were, she worried about her mother and her job. Terri rarely exhibited the side of her that must have trembled with worry for her sister, mother, their economic survival and her job security. For one so young, these were too many balls to keep in the air. It wasn't in her nature to express these concerns, but they were noticeably evident in the lines etched into her brow, in hazel eyes gazing into the distance, and in the biting of her fingernails. I ached for her. I knew she drew comfort from confiding in my daughter. I only hoped that their conversations helped relieve some of her pressures.

Our own private talks outside Sylvia's room gave me a mental picture of what home life with Sylvia had become. From bits and pieces of conversation, I learned that when Sylvia was well, Terri enjoyed sisterly companionship as well as financial support from Sylvia's sharing in the household expenses. Sylvia could be a buddy, fun to hang around with and an active partner in the life they'd made without their father.

On the other hand, when unwell, Sylvia became shrouded in melancholy. She became another self—one that was sleepy, listless, withdrawn and impatient to the point of tears. This seesawing of moods had shown prior to surgery. Terri had caught a glimpse of it again just before this recent hospitalization. She worried about what it might mean. I tried to reassure her that, with the readjustment of meds, Sylvia might finally be on her way back to good health.

"Maybe this'll be the last time you have to make the trip over here, *mija*. Let's keep our fingers crossed." I said it firmly, hoping to lift Terri's spirits as well as my own.

It was almost dinner time when I turned to Terri and Cynthia. "I think I'll go home now." I said to Cynthia, "What about you, *mija*? Are you staying until your *tia* gets here?"

"Yeah, Mom. I'll wait with Terri. Maybe we'll go get something to eat after *tia* comes. If they go to Chu's, I might stop by at Tim and Kim's for a while." They were close friends who also knew Sylvia. She'd attended high school with them.

"Yeah, that's a good idea, *mija*. I'll see you whenever you get in."

As it turned out, Maggie arrived shortly after I left, and she and the girls stayed until visiting hours were over.

The following Sunday, the girls, my *comadre* and I took turns visiting with Sylvia most of the day. Terri had decided to stick with Cynthia and slept at our place while her mom stayed with her sister. On Monday morning, as Terri left for the hospital and I for work, I called to her before she went out the door. "I'll come by after work, *mija*. About five-thirty. I'll call you around noon to find out if the test results are back, okay?"

"That's fine, *tia*. See you later."

As promised, I called Sylvia's room on my lunch hour. When Terri answered, I asked, "Well?"

"She should be on her way back from the biopsy any minute now. She looked better when she left, but I don't know, *tia*..." Terri's tired voice trailed off.

"Okay, *mija*, I'll call you later when you know something more definite, say, in a couple of hours or so. In the meantime, if Dr. Amend talks to you, will you call me at the office, please?" Dr. Amend was Sylvia's lead physician and had been for many years.

"Sure, *tia*. Thanks for calling."

I knew my *comadre* was also in the room. It was hard for us to speak at times like this because of the common fears flowing between us, or so I felt. While at the time we might talk about the kids or other family matters, our thoughts were really on Sylvia. Even as we made polite conversation, we knew none of it mattered. And our real thoughts wouldn't convert to verbal expression. By unspoken, mutual consent we were often silent together; mothers with unspoken fears and boundless hope. It seemed so incredibly cruel that she should have to go through such anxiety. Wasn't losing Mando enough? How much more could she bear? I often wondered.

Happily, when I called the hospital later in the afternoon, good news greeted me! Terri's voice exuded cheerfulness.

"Well, her creatinine is coming down, and the biopsy shows that the kidney is not in rejection. Isn't that good news, *tia*?" Terri could hardly catch her breath. "So it looks like they just have to readjust the meds again, that's all."

My own breath caught. "Hallelujah!" I screamed and started to laugh, giddy with relief. "I knew it'd be all right. Oh, what super news, *mija*. Ask her if there's anything she wants me to bring her tonight. Burritos? A hamburger? Milkshake?"

I could hear Terri repeating my offer and heard Sylvia's soft response in the background, "No, nothing. Thanks."

"Did you hear that, *tia*? Missy doesn't want a thing!" The welcomed taunting attitude was back in Terri's voice.

Terri and Maggie left the hospital for Stockton about mid-afternoon that Monday to try and beat the Interstate 680 commuter traffic, which can only be described as the commute from hell. By this time they knew that Sylvia would remain at the hospital for a couple of days while her adjusted meds kicked in, then stay with me for a day or so before returning home. As usual, Cynthia, her other cousins and relatives plus friends and I would keep Sylvia company at the hospital and take her the treats she often craved.

About five o'clock that day, I left my office for the all-too-familiar ninth floor's KTU (kidney transplant unit). Using the parking lot on a daily basis could become expensive, so I'd developed a pattern of scouting for empty street parking spots close to the hospital. Others were doing the same thing. As a result, I would end up circling the medical complex several times before finding a car exiting a coveted site or discovering a recently abandoned spot. If I was out of luck, the parking lot was the only alternative. Getting from there across the street to the right hospital floor meant the usual twists and turns from elevators to street crossing, up ascending staircases, descending staircases and endless corridors. But by this time, I could navigate the maze in my sleep. On this particular evening, I floated to Sylvia's room.

"Hi, *mija*. How ya doing?" I rushed to peck her forehead.

Relief bathed her face. "Much better, *nina*. I feel so silly. All that worry and trouble, and it's only a med adjustment." She shook her head as she pushed her dinner tray away. "That stuff was awful. I ate the Jell-O, though. Can't believe I actually liked it. How are YOU doing, *nina*? Geez, you look nice."

She always told me I looked nice. Actually, at the time I felt that odd sense of tiredness that overtakes one after a worry has been lifted. Letting go of fretting leaves you exhausted.

"I hear the results of the biopsy were good, huh? They're taking you off the 'K' medicine, whatever that is, and putting you back on the cyclosporine, which should do the trick. Right?"

She gave me the correct name of the "K" medication, which promptly went out of my head, and added, "Yeah, that's what they tell me."

"Boy, what a relief, huh, *mija*?"

We chatted, watched the evening news and caught up on the latest buzz about family and friends. Her energy level was rising and her usual mental sharpness returning—both comforting signs. After *Wheel of Fortune* finished, I said, "Well, I'm off, *mija*. I'll be back tomorrow. Anything you want me to bring?"

"Will you ask Cindy to send me some shampoo and conditioner, please? I can't believe I came without it. It felt soooo good to take a shower today, but I used regular hand soap on my hair and I can feel it. Yuck." She ran her fingers through the length of her hair, making a face.

"Sure." I gave her a loud smack on the cheek and said, "Be good and sleep tight."

I imagined that before long things would be back on course. In fact, I was confident they would be. But this latest occurrence showed that even a successful transplant is not without worrisome episodes. It's not unusual to experience such incidences until the right balance of medications and dosages is established. It's part and parcel of the process during the first months after surgery for an organ recipient. It helps to remember that even with the erratic ups and downs involved, it's still miles ahead of the alternative.

In our case, during such times the value of the KTU was immeasurable. The staff were dedicated and highly effective. They propped spirits up and buoyed our hopes without giving false expectations. They never failed to impart the feeling that they truly cared. To this day, I can't thank or praise them enough.

By Saturday, Sylvia's creatinine and other numbers had dropped to acceptable levels, and we were able to bring her to San Bruno. The following day happened to be Mother's Day, and Cynthia had planned her usual special brunch for me and her *tias*, my sisters. My Joe was working a computer show at Moscone Center that day and couldn't join us.

My sisters had known Sylvia from the time she was a tiny tot and were well aware of her place in my family's life. The youngest, Betty, couldn't come that Sunday. But when Esther, Elvie and Beatriz arrived at ten-thirty in the morning, they greeted Sylvia like a niece of their own. I knew they were genuinely pleased to see her. They inquired about her health and about Maggie, whom they also knew well.

The "girls" (as my sisters and I refer to ourselves) and Sylvia, Cynthia and I were all talking a mile a minute. We sipped our mimosas, enjoying the luxury of being pampered. Cynthia scurried to get things on the beautifully set table. Sylvia sat on the sofa with a drink of water and laughed along with us as we shared stories. We find a lot of humor in sharing the funny things we do or that happen to us. Elvie's stories are always the best and funniest.

Elvie, one of the twins, worked for the Legal Aid Society in Redwood City for almost twenty years. She started out as a receptionist and later assumed additional responsibilities. As might be expected, she was very nervous on her first day on the job. Her duties were to answer phones, greet clients, announce the arrival of the clients to the attorney they'd come to see, and then walk them back to that attorney's office. One of the first clients to walk in on that fateful day was a Mr. Moran. Elvie notified the proper attorney and accompanied Mr. Moran to the correct office. Opening the door, she announced the client. "Mr. Moron here to see you."

With great indignation, the client corrected her. "That's Mr. Moran!"

Mortified, Elvie skulked out of the office and returned to the front desk. Fully expecting to be chastised for her blunder, she was relieved when nothing was said. When she told us about it, we literally howled. We all took turns making fun of ourselves and of each other, something we enjoy doing to this day. For whatever reason, no matter how hard the rest of us try, Elvie's escapades outshine the rest of ours.

Eventually, Cynthia proudly announced, "Okay, you can sit down now."

Our eyes widened as we viewed the table. There were small, individual spinach and mushroom quiches, perfectly-browned sausages, muffins, a huge bowlful of picture-perfect strawberries, whipped cream, scrumptious pastries, juices and a carafe of fresh coffee.

"Wow!" Esther, the other twin, exclaimed.

Middle sister Beatriz blinked at the spread and oohed and ahhed, raising her brows in unmistakable approval. I was too busy smiling with pride to comment.

"Aren't you glad I had a daughter?" I teased my twin sisters, who both had sons.

We chuckled while passing the platters around. I was surprised that Sylvia remained on the sofa. Instead of joining us, she excused herself. "I'm going up to take a little nap before I take off. It was so nice to see all of you."

As if on cue, all said, "Oh. Are you sure you don't want anything?"

"No, not now. Maybe later." She turned and went upstairs.

I quickly said, "Sure, *mija*. Close the door. If we make too much noise, holler. We'll try and save you some of these fabulous goodies."

Actually, there was enough food on the table to feed twice our number. Even though Sylvia wasn't actually sitting at the table with us, I still sensed her presence upstairs and was pleased to have her there. It seemed fitting that we should share this particular Mother's Day.

For two hours we ate, generously complimenting our hostess. Because Cynthia and I had a date for three o'clock that afternoon, which the girls were aware of, they left before two o'clock. Several weeks beforehand, I'd purchased tickets for Cynthia and me to attend the matinee performance of *Hello Dolly* with Carol Channing playing at the city's Orpheum Theatre. My daughter is an ardent fan of Carol Channing, especially in her role as Dolly.

As I was freshening up in the downstairs bathroom, Sylvia appeared. The door was open and she came in, approaching me with outstretched arms.

"I'm on my way, *nina*. Hope you and the brat enjoy the play."

Her silky hair was brushed up in a ponytail. A touch of lip gloss gave her a rosy look. I squeezed her tightly. "You're okay driving back? Let me fix you a goodie bag for the ride." She certainly looked refreshed and back to her old self.

"Oh, no thanks, *nina*. I had some toast earlier. No problem. I'm going to put my stuff in the car. Be right back."

I agreed that she seemed well enough for the drive to Stockton, and it was obvious that she was anxious to get home to her own mother on this special day. She was also planning to go to work the following morning, so I was convinced that she really did feel good. When she returned, she retrieved her medicines from Cynthia's bedroom, then headed down the stairs to the front door. All seemed beautifully normal.

"Thank you again, *nina*." She gave me another embrace.

"*Mija*, I'm always glad to have you. Next time make it just a regular visit, okay?"

"I hope so." She gave me a look of frustration and shook her head, although her eyes were smiling.

As if to reassure me, she added, "I'm fine, really. I like driving, and it's the middle of the day, so there shouldn't be much traffic. I'll do the slow lane, take my time, play my tapes. No sweat. I prefer going slow anyway."

"Okay, that's good. Call when you get home, please." The three of us walked out the front door.

She waved as she climbed into her grey Nissan. "Enjoy Carol Channing!" she called out from the open car window as she passed us.

We watched her drive off, smiling and waving as she coasted down the short street. Lost in our own thoughts, we stood watching the car as it disappeared around the corner. Then, without expressing our disquieting concerns, for fear, perhaps, that their utterance might make them come true, we silently got into my car and drove to the matinee. That Mother's Day was the last time we saw Sylvia up and about.

18

The Last Hospital Stay

On Saturday, May 20th, Terri brought Sylvia back to the hospital. Sylvia had developed a sinus infection days earlier. She'd gone to her local doctor, who'd prescribed an antibiotic. For some reason, Sylvia didn't respond to the prescription and became increasingly sicker. Eventually, she was so weak that Maggie and Terri had to practically carry her into the car. The news was crushing.

The immunosuppressants essential to Sylvia on a daily basis may have contributed to the ineffectiveness of the medication she'd received. To this day, we're not sure exactly what happened, but whatever the cause, she was experiencing another setback. From what we could gather from Terri, this one was worse than the last.

I'd gotten the news late that evening, and of course, first thing in the morning both Cynthia and I rushed to UCSF. We said very little on the drive up. We knew what floor to go to and headed in that direction. At the nurse's station, we asked for Sylvia's room and hurried toward it.

My *comadre* sat in the corner, staring blankly out the window. Sylvia lay motionless beneath the rumpled covers of her bed, snoring softly. Her labored breathing raised and lowered the thin blankets. A negative mood permeated the room. I had to fend off its disheartening assault before I greeted Maggie.

"*Comadre.*" I hugged her and whispered, not wanting to wake Sylvia.

My *comadre* could barely muster a response. "Hi, *comadre.*"

Cynthia embraced her *tia*. Sylvia, stirred by our voices, turned toward us. At the sight of me, she grimaced, covered her face and cried.

"Oh, *nina*. I'm so sorry. So sorry. I've let everyone down." Her sobs were wrenching. Desolation overwhelmed her.

I sat on the bed beside her. "*Mija*, don't. It'll be all right. You'll see. You haven't ever let me down. It's just another temporary setback. I think that darn sinus infection just got the best of you. They'll fix it. Don't worry, *mija*, it'll be all right."

She was convulsed with grief and torment. It shook me to the core. For the first time, I feared for her and for us. I wouldn't believe that the situation could be as severe as Sylvia felt it to be. I told myself her outburst was due to the culmination of weeks of frustration. It had to be. From the disappointing false starts, her tiredness, and a misplaced sense of self-reproach. For Sylvia, her existence had turned into chronic affliction and burden to her family.

She continued to sob, apologizing all the while. The depth of her distress was frightening. I stayed focused on the infection and its resolution. I refused to be disheartened. But it was the first time I'd ever seen her so dejected and inconsolable. No trace of her inner angel peered through. How strange not to see the fighting spirit. It wasn't the same Sylvia.

"I don't know what's the matter with me," she bawled. "I just don't feel good anymore." Between sobs, she kept repeating, "I'm so sorry."

"Shhh, it's okay, *mija*. You know it's going to be okay. They'll find out what the trouble is and make it better. Let's not get impatient." How false my own words sounded, yet I felt the need to say something. I couldn't stand the fact that she was blaming herself for being ill. Her desperation was alarming. It took a lot of self-control to smother my fears. I stifled a surging panic.

"Where does it hurt?" I asked.

"I have a horrible headache. And my chest, it hurts to breathe." She touched her ribcage and rested her hand upon it, weeping all the while.

I turned to Maggie. "What do the doctors say?"

Maggie struggled to find her voice. She finally said, "We don't know yet. It's the weekend, and tomorrow, Monday, Dr. Amend will be here to see her. For now, they're just monitoring her. Because she's complaining about her chest, they took some X-rays. They've given her something for the headache, but it doesn't seem to help. I just don't know, *comadre*..." Her voice faded away as she turned to stare back out the window.

When I gazed into *comadre's* eyes, they were dry of tears. Her face was pinched with worry. *How much more can she take?* I asked myself.

A nurse came. Silently, she wrote something into the chart hooked at the end of the bed. For the first time, I noticed that Sylvia had an oxygen tube in her nose, and I asked the nurse, "Is the oxygen because of the sinus infection?"

She nodded, then concentrated on the chart entries. She was one of the nurses who'd previously taken care of Sylvia. She, too, seemed unnaturally quiet. I turned my attention back to my godchild. Patting her hand, I noticed that they'd inserted a tube for the dialysis treatment. It was a discouraging sign. Why would a sinus infection require dialysis? Sylvia must have noticed the look on my face.

"I'm having dialysis tomorrow," she explained. "Just a precaution, *nina*. To take the strain off my kidney. I'll also have another biopsy. Thank God they're better than they used to be." Her voice was husky, but she was calmer as she dabbed her eyes with a tissue.

"Boy," I said, trying to soften the mood. "Remember the first one you had thirteen years ago? You swore you'd never have another one again. I'm so glad they've improved and that you don't mind them anymore. So, what's with the sinus infection? What are they doing about that?"

I slid onto the chair next to her bed and tried to look relaxed.

"Oh, I don't know, *nina*. I thought my allergies were acting up. But when the headaches got so bad, I went to see the doctor. It turned out to be my sinuses. He prescribed some medicine. It didn't seem to help, and I got so weak..." Her words tapered off. Tears fell again.

"I'm so sorry," she whispered. "We're supposed to be helping you, our parents, not you helping us." Where had this heavy dose of guilt come from? It was so unlike Sylvia.

I assumed she felt responsible for not being healthy enough and worrying her mother with her repeated visits to the hospital. This realization pierced me to the core. Even worse, her eyes mirrored a painful sense of being a burden. Right or wrong, Mexican mothers do look to their daughters for support, comfort and solace. It's inculcated into our culture. Having a daughter is a kind of insurance that someone will look after us in our old age. Sons are caring, but possible interference from the daughter-in-law always looms in the background. For that reason, the daughter and mother relationship is traditionally more co-dependent. Other cultures also rely on daughters to care for the parents.

It was this tradition that Sylvia felt she wasn't living up to. It had never occurred to me that it bothered her so much. It wasn't until that day that I realized how devastating this sense of failure was. It lay like a granite boulder on her soul, breaking her heart and shattering her spirit. It must have been gnawing at her for a long time until the emotion could no longer contain the guilt.

"*Mija, mija*, it's all right. It's not your fault. You're going to get better, you'll see. They've fixed you up before, haven't they? Give them a chance to get to the bottom of the problem, and it'll be okay again. Shhh, don't worry so."

I reached over to touch her leg. "*Mija*, there aren't any limits for our children, you know that. When you need, we automatically respond without thought. That's what we're here for, to help one another. I'm sure your mom and Terri don't feel you're a bother. They're just anxious for you to get the help you need, and nothing else matters. Don't let such thoughts get you down, *mija*."

"But *nina*. She and Terri almost had to carry me into the car. Actually carry me!" The memory pained her. It seemed like the ultimate degradation, too severe an indignity to forget. I'd never seen Sylvia so totally despondent, and that, more than her condition, greatly worried me.

I got up to so I could hold her close, silently hugging and rocking her back and forth in my arms. Shortly, her shudders subsided and her tears stopped.

"We can't give up now, *mija*. We've come too far. Don't get impatient, please." Easy for me to say, I thought, when I was up and about. "Tomorrow they'll make sure your kidney's all right and then go from there. Hey! Have you been eating enough chocolate? Maybe that's the problem."

I pulled out a small packet of Hershey Kisses from my purse and placed them on the bed tray. "Just in case you need a shot," I said.

Her giggle was encouraging. She became more relaxed, breathing naturally and ready for another nap. We stayed several hours, then left to await what the next day would bring.

On Monday, I called her room from the office to see if there was anything she wanted me to take when I stopped by after work. No one answered. A bit later, I called her room again, and still no answer. The third time, I called the nurses' station and was told, "Oh, Sylvia Zertuche has been moved to the cardiac unit on the tenth floor."

"The cardiac unit!" I barked. "Why?"

"You'll have to check with the nurses' station there," she said. "Let me transfer you."

The nurse in the cardiac unit said that while Sylvia had been in dialysis that morning, her blood pressure had dropped dramatically, making her feel faint. They thought the infection might have been too much of a strain on her heart, so they had placed her in the cardiac unit as a precautionary measure.

I could hardly wait to get to the hospital. Normally, crossing the Golden Gate Bridge from the Marin side to the city never ceases to take my breath away. The Pacific Ocean on one side of the span and the San Francisco Bay on the other are spectacular in bright sunlight, misty fog or driving rain, as is the city's skyline with its familiar landmarks. The massive citadel of a rock now housing the ruins of what was once Alcatraz prison adds to the dramatic view. Freighters, tankers, sailboats, barges, yachts, cruise ships—all like miniature toys in the enormous bay—stream by on their way to the docks or out toward the Farrallones, gate to the Pacific. In either direction, they adorn the waterway and arouse a mental excitement of past adventures featuring Portola, Cabrillo, Balboa, Sir Francis Drake, and the successive hordes that followed their dreams sailing into the harbor.

But that day, I don't even remember crossing the bridge. I don't remember parking the car. I just found myself striding down the tenth floor hallway.

Maggie, like one of the fixtures, was there. I could only imagine her anguish. She stood by the bedside and barely mustered a smile when I entered the room.

"Hi, *comadre*," she said.

Unspoken fears lay heavy in the air. Not voicing them shielded us from additional heartache and dread. For the moment, we chose silence as the only comfort available. I looked at the oxygen tubes and the still form of my godchild as she slept on the cranked-up bed. Eventually, I asked, "*Comadre*. How are you?" Such an inane comment.

A weary voice answered, "Oh, fine."

"So, I hear this is just a precaution," I said.

"That's what they tell us," Maggie said.

More silence. Maggie turned her head from the bed toward the window and gazed far into the billowed gray of descending fog. I walked out to the nurses' station and requested that Sylvia's nurse stop by to speak with us when she had a chance. About fifteen minutes later, a nurse entered the room.

"I'm not Sylvia's regular nurse, but I'm going to take her vitals and jot them down."

As she spoke, she grabbed the blood pressure bag from its hook behind the back of the bed and wrapped it around Sylvia's forearm. The red binder containing Sylvia's chart was spread across the sink. The nurse noted down her readings of blood pressure, temperature, etc. Then she snapped the plastic clothespin-type apparatus that measured the oxygen levels in the blood off Sylvia's finger, tapped it and reapplied it. This is the kind of thing that flashes red lights in the minds of patients' families regardless of how routine it may actually be.

"I'm not getting much of a reading," she muttered to herself. Sylvia awoke when the nurse started taking her vital signs. The nurse asked, "Sylvia, can you give me a cough?"

Sylvia made a weak attempt to cough.

"Come on, dear. Do a little better for me."

Sylvia grabbed the side bar to brace herself and tried again. This time the effort developed into a coughing spasm—a deep, dry, wracking spell that caused her to clutch her side in pain.

With difficulty, she whispered, "Oh, it hurts when I cough. They think I popped a rib…" She was interrupted by another coughing fit.

"That's all right. Take it easy now." The nurse patted Sylvia's shoulder. After a moment, she asked, "You okay? Want some water? How about a little sip?" She filled a glass with some water and gently raised it to Sylvia's lips.

I didn't like the worried look on the nurse's face, or was it just my imagination? The coughing subsided and Sylvia sank back into the pillows, closing her eyes, wearied to exhaustion. The nurse left, commenting to Maggie and me, "Her regular nurse will be in to see you before too long."

Maggie stared at her daughter, and for a moment, her features reminded me of Michelangelo's *Pieta*. Soon she returned to her reverie beyond the opaqueness of the window. I sat in the chair at the foot of the bed, at a loss to understand what was happening to Sylvia. It's difficult to be comforting when one doesn't understand. I touched Sylvia's leg. "What hurts when you're not coughing, *mija*?"

"If I'm quiet, nothing does. It's just that I'm so very tired. I don't think I've ever been so tired. I'm okay if I don't cough. It's this rib. They think I've popped it from so much coughing. It's really sore and hurts like mad when I do cough." She spoke in breathy gasps with her eyes closed, her head sideways on the pillow.

When her regular nurse came in, I pounced on her. "I had a telephone request for Dr. Amend to call me this afternoon and didn't hear from him. I'd like to know what the status is here. Why is she in the cardiac unit?" I made every attempt to keep my voice moderated, but some of my anxiety-driven anger came through.

Being professional and having encountered frightened relatives before, she calmly nodded to me, as if saying she'd attend to me in a moment. Directing her attention to Sylvia, she approached her with a wonderful smile.

"Hi! How're you doing? Coughing hurts, doesn't it?" She rubbed Sylvia's arm sympathetically, which got a nod from her patient.

Turning to me, she explained, "While she was having dialysis this morning, she almost fainted and her blood pressure dropped. That can cause a real strain on the heart, so she's here for observation purposes to make sure her blood pressure recovers and to be monitored in general. In this unit, we have someone looking at the screens constantly. Dr. Amend feels this is where she needs to be at the moment."

"Then nothing's wrong with her heart? She's not in danger of an impending heart attack or anything like that?" I asked.

"No, just making sure everything is stable," she said patiently as she grabbed the red binder to review its notations.

I turned to my *comadre*, who was nodding her head with relief. "Oh, that's wonderful. Thank you, thank you."

The nurse added, as if for confirmation, "And Dr. Amend said that the kidney is a little lazy, but that the new medication should re-energize it in a few days." Again she turned to Sylvia. "There, there. It's all right." As she patted Sylvia's legs, she also tucked her in, fluffed up her pillows and adjusted the oxygen tubes. This brought an audible sigh from Sylvia, and no further coughing was heard during the remainder of our stay.

Maggie's attention was back in the room. Some of the tiredness left her voice as we talked quietly about where she was staying, how long, and who was taking care of her grandson during her absence. She said she'd already had dinner, but I wondered if that was true. I offered to take her home around eight o'clock. We left a quiet, snoozing Sylvia in the room, and it appeared that she was going to sleep the whole night through without any difficulty. That lightened our moods.

When we reached the in-laws' house in South City where Maggie was staying, I asked her, "Do you want me to pick you up in the morning? About seven-thirty? I can drop you off at the hospital and go to work from there."

"Yes, *comadre*. I'll be ready. *Gracias*."

I was ten minutes late the following morning, and Maggie scurried out of the house before I could beep the horn. Obviously, she'd been watching for me from the glass-paned porch.

I apologized in Spanish. "Sorry I'm late, *comadre*. The sheets stuck to me this morning." That's a favorite saying inherited from my grandmother, who had a lot of experience with my reluctance to get up during my school days. It sounds cuter in Spanish than it does in English.

Commuter traffic on Sunset Drive was the usual ordeal. Eventually, we were in front of the hospital vying for a drop-off space.

"I'll come by about six o'clock to visit and take you home, *comadre*. Give her a kiss for me. Be sure and get some food, okay?"

It was a drizzly Tuesday. I watched Maggie walk away, climb the entrance stairs and enter the building. The sense of purpose, determination, and all the fortitude she could muster showed in her posture, the way she walked. She was trying to stay strong. I watched her enter the familiar institution that housed her daughter and which had refused to relinquish her for too long. It reminded me of my early divorce distress. Life weighs heavily when it takes every ounce of energy and stamina to remain functional. Focusing becomes impossible. But this was infinitely worse for my *comadre*. Nothing equals the terror of having your child in jeopardy. Perhaps today would be a good day for both mother and daughter.

As it turned out, Tuesday was a repeat of the preceding day. So was Wednesday. Then it was Thursday. On schedule, I called the hospital about mid-afternoon from work to see if there was something I could bring before dropping by. There was no answer from Sylvia's room. I called the nurses' station and was informed that Sylvia was now in the intensive care unit. Hanging up the phone, I gathered my things together.

"John, Sylvia's in ICU. I've got to go."

Fortunately, my boss was extremely understanding and patient during this time. He shot me a concerned look. "How come? I thought she was getting better."

"I don't know. I didn't speak with Maggie. I'll call you later and let you know what's going on." I hurried out the door.

19

Antibiotic Cocktails

At the hospital I found Maggie with Michelle, our niece who worked at UC as an administrative assistant. There was a special bond between them that had started from Michelle's orphaned babyhood. Now she was in her early twenties and slender to the point of being almost skinny. She moved her five foot, six inch frame gracefully, as if the amount of time it took to reach a spot didn't matter. Her dark brown eyes matched the shade of her naturally curly hair and blended well with her doe-like skin. Even though Michelle had been brought up by Serjio and Josie, her mother's sister, Michelle loved Maggie like a second mom.

They were sitting, much like mother and daughter, in the ICU waiting room, just outside the double doors that housed the more critical patients. When Maggie spotted me, tears trickled down her cheeks as she shook her head slowly from side to side. It was a forlorn gesture. I hugged her and Michelle before sitting down next to my *comadre*.

"So, what do they say?" I whispered.

Maggie lowered the tissue from her face, sighed and repeated by rote what the doctors had said.

"It seems that she now has pneumonia. It showed up yesterday when they took the chest x-rays. Dr. Amend wants her here where she can be carefully watched. She's on a breathing machine so her lungs don't have to work too hard." She tried to sound hopeful that this was a newly discovered conduit towards the path to recovery. She added, "She's getting more antibiotics. You want to go in to see her?" Turning to Michelle, she said, "*Mija*, why don't you go pick up your things in your office and meet us in here later, after you get off of work?" I knew Michelle hadn't wanted to leave her *tia* alone, and now that I was here with her, she agreed to go back to her office.

Nothing could have kept me out of ICU. Without replying to Maggie's request, I stood and both of us headed toward the pair of metal doors. When we pressed the plaque on the wall, the doors swooshed inward to reveal a different world of quiet movement, hushed tones, and higher ratios of nurses to patients. I followed her in. We promptly turned right into the first cubicle.

As practiced as I'd become at masking difficult emotions, the sight of Sylvia caught me completely off guard. My mind wanted to scream, "This can't be her!" My brain knew otherwise, but my heart must have accepted the harsh reality, for it sickened me down to my stomach. I approached the high bed silently and touched the sheeted lump of her thigh. Forcing myself not to cry, I spoke to her.

Was it possible that this was the infant I'd cradled over the baptismal font? The child I'd delighted in? The young woman I'd given a part of myself to? How could this be? She shouldn't have nine bags of fluids attached to her or multitudes of lines exiting her body like tangled tentacles. A colorful monitor flashed overhead with numbers graphing erratic activity. A ventilator was doing her breathing. She was too still, too quiet. I struggled against the ugliness of the reality; ashamed that I wasn't as brave as my *comadre*.

"Hi, *mija*. It's *nina*." I went on, "So, you've got a touch of pneumonia now." Like she hadn't heard this before. Did I imagine that she nodded? Leaning over the bed railing, I stroked her hand. In soothing tones I pleaded, "Relax, *mija*. Just relax and let the medicines take their course. Let the machine do your breathing so you can get better soon. We'll be here, you know that."

I could see she was heavily sedated. Nurses always encourage people to talk to sedated or unconscious patients, and I continued with more talk, hoping my words were filtering through. I kept my hand on her forehead, stroking the dark, glossy braids and caressing her cheeks. I refused to see the swollen body, visualizing instead the svelte, smiling, bright-eyed *mija* that I knew was hidden within.

Her nose was the only part of her that retained its original shape. It remained perfect even with the oxygen tubes inserted in her nostrils. I'd always loved her pert nose, probably because I'd always hated my own pudgy one. Her mouth was stuffed with an apparatus that held her tongue to prevent its rolling back. The large amount of fluid intake had caused swelling to every part of her being, and a huge double chin lay across her throat. Hoses connected her to the artificial breathing machine.

Someone had braided her lush, shiny hair into a long rope and daintily arranged it atop her head. The white scallops of the hair-tie were an incongruous decoration, but revealed the level of care. It was definitely Maggie's touch, and so in keeping with Sylvia's habit of keeping her hair perfectly groomed.

For the first time my spirit faltered. I was truly frightened. *Don't panic, stay calm. She'll bounce back again; she has to.* I repeated the thoughts over and over.

My soft words poured out. They were just as much for my benefit as for hers. Alarmed at feeling so helpless, at what her transfer into this unit really signified, at the panicky thoughts racing through me, I fought to remain optimistic. Somewhere there had to be a seed of hope. Surely, this situation would be turned around.

Snatches of conversation between Sylvia and me were spaced in intervals. My *comadre* seemed out of words. After a while, Michelle rejoined us, and her presence was consoling to both of us. The cubicle went quiet as we inwardly withdrew. If you don't voice your fears, maybe they won't materialize.

Seeking distraction, I scanned the glassed-in cubicle and the surroundings. In front of every ICU room was a tall, podium-type desk with a swivel chair for that room's nurse. From there she observed the monitor, heard the dinging generated from an empty fluid bag, watched the ventilator-induced breathing of her patient, jotted down observations, explained those notes to the parade of specialists drifting in and out,

209

answered phones and hovered protectively over visitors, especially family. These angels in white routinely perform and witness miracles with little acknowledgment. They're joyous in victory, resigned in defeat, and resilient enough to overcome the effects of seeing death on such a regular basis.

I imagine no amount of training can shield anyone from exposure to the deep emotions these nurses encountered. Yet they remained resolute in providing the care so vital to all their patients. Working twelve-hour shifts, ICU nurses are perhaps the most intense of all caregivers. Observing them in action as they flitted quietly about was an eye-opening glimpse into their special vocation. We had never appreciated or needed them more. Sylvia was in the best possible hands, and we drew what strength we could from that.

Nearby, Sylvia's day nurse was briefing the evening nurse. It was the changing of the guard, and I knew the briefing on Sylvia's condition would be thorough. I strained to hear.

"One hundred percent on the ventilator... low pressure... resistant... portable dialysis... oxygenation level slightly better..." I tried to glean every morsel of information in case they told each other things they hadn't told us. Under normal circumstances, I would have realized that they were too well trained for such amateurish attempts to work.

When we'd been there over an hour, the evening nurse was comfortably transitioned. When she came into our cubicle, I asked her about the numbers on the monitor.

"What's the upper red figure?"

She responded that it was the pulse.

"I know that the yellow numbers are the systolic and diastolic numbers of her blood pressure, but what about the number off to the side of them?"

She explained that it was the oxygenation level. The flickering graphs seemed like endless, repetitious patterns of measurements that I'd never heard of and have since forgotten. I focused on the blood pressure numbers, which were below normal. Every time they jumped up a notch, I pointed it out to my *comadre* and Michelle. I remember holding my breath between changes. Forty-three is not a terrific number when associated with blood pressure, yet it was an improvement. Later that evening, the numbers inched higher—into the seventies—and we became greatly encouraged. Our thoughts were that the worst had to be over.

The nurse, observing my obsession with the numbers on the monitor, cautioned, "You know, that data is just a part of the total, overall condition. Don't pay too much attention to the shifting numbers. It's when they make dramatic drops or increases that they really tell us something."

Her gentle cautioning may have been an attempt to prepare us for the inevitable. But her experience was no match for our optimism. I remember thinking that she should have been more positive. She should have been relishing the moment when she would see how Sylvia would make a complete turnaround and release her space for a more critical patient. Then she'd realize how unnecessarily doubtful she'd been.

We left ICU about ten o'clock. Though tired, we were comfortable knowing that Sylvia had stabilized. Or so we thought.

The next day was the Saturday morning of Memorial Day weekend. Don picked me up to take me to the hospital. When we arrived, we found Cynthia, Michelle and Maggie talking with Dr. Amend in the ICU waiting room. Furnished with a comfortable sofa, club chairs, a coffee table with magazines, and a television set, it was meant to ease lengthy, precarious hours. Everyone looked somber, most especially Dr. Amend. We were just in time to join the start of the conference and eagerly sat down to hear the latest diagnosis.

He addressed himself mainly to Maggie. "She's a very sick girl. In addition to the pneumonia, she has a viral infection and a bacterial infection in her lungs. We've introduced an aggressive antibiotic program, but it could take several days before we see any results. I think it's beginning to get under control, though." He unclasped his hands and slapped them on his thighs. "We'll continue to keep her sedated so that she doesn't exert herself in any way. The nurses tell me that she resists their attempts to move her or change an intravenous line, so we've increased the narcotic dosage to keep her body immobile. It'll keep her body from working too hard. But remember, she still may be able to hear you, so keep on talking to her. As soon as we can, we'll cut back on it. But for now, it's best for her to be as sedated as possible."

At one point, he elaborated on the "cocktail" of antibiotics. The strategy behind administering the combination of various infection fighters he called cocktails represented a more aggressive tactic. One of the objectives was to prevent Sylvia's body from poisoning itself by becoming too acidic, a natural defense mechanism against infection. As for me, I listened to what I wished to hear, selectively plucking out only the positive words from his overall report. I liked my own version of reality better.

Dr. Amend was sitting on an ottoman in front of Maggie while the rest of us formed a semi-circle around him. She had listened too well. Uncharacteristically, she lashed out at him. "You promised me she'd get better! You said she would!" She pointed her finger accusingly in his face before gagging on her muffled sobs. Grief poured into the cupped hands, a deluge long bottled up. She shielded us from the torment on her face.

Dr. Amend flinched as if visibly struck, then replied, "We're trying, Maggie. Really we are. We're doing everything possible that can be done. She has heart specialists, respiratory specialists, nephrologists, technicians and the best nurses all around her. You know I'm keeping a close eye on her. She's very special to me." His tone pleaded for understanding while his arm reached out to pat her on the shoulder. "We've been through a lot these last years, Maggie. We'll get through this, too."

Maggie and Sylvia had always referred to both Dr. Vicente and Dr. Amend in the most reverent of terms since the beginning of Sylvia's illness. These doctors were superhuman beings, above ordinary physicians, imbued with infallibility and compassionate in their ministrations. Their word was the embodiment of science, which made them close to being venerated in Maggie's and, at one time, in Mando's eyes. To witness Maggie's disillusionment was astonishing. It surprised us, but we understood. To Dr. Amend's credit, he heard only the frightened words of a mother.

He rose slowly, pausing momentarily for either our questions or additional accusations. When neither Maggie nor I spoke, he left.

I sat next to Maggie, my arm around her. I was as bewildered as she and equally helpless. Maggie wept, and the sound pierced our hearts. Her anguish was heart-rending. That's when I admitted to being afraid. There was nothing to say. We'd heard first-hand how serious Sylvia's condition was, and there was nothing we could do about it. Hope eluded us as we fought against the sin of all sins, despair.

Such moments suspend time. At some point, Maggie calmed herself and was the first to return to the present. She stood up straight, folded her arms against her bosom and walked toward the inner sanctum that isolated her daughter. There was a taut quality about her that made me wonder if she were about to snap. Who'd blame her?

I hadn't seen Sylvia as yet, so I followed my *comadre* through the ICU doors, entering Sylvia's cubicle with my usual greeting. "Hi, *mija*, it's *nina.*"

Grasping at the possibility that my words reached some deep, unknown reservoir of consciousness, I rambled on. "The reason you can't move, *mija*, is that the doctors want to keep you as relaxed as possible to allow the ventilator to breathe for you so your lungs recuperate. Don't let that worry you. You'll be able to move all you want once this infection clears up." Patting the coverlet smooth, I went on. "For now, *mija*, rest and get better. When they come to move you, let them. Don't use up any precious energy. Save it to get better. We need you to get well, and we're going to stay until you do. We're right here, *mija*, don't be afraid. We love you so much."

My hand automatically stroked her forehead. Perhaps she could feel my touch. "Let my love heal you," I prayed.

Maggie sat on a chair on the other side of the bed, gently massaging Sylvia's hand and uttering words that might plant the necessary resolve within her daughter. It struck me that her soft mumblings were not unlike the little private conversations a mother has with her newborn infant. In our hearts, our children are always our precious infants.

Another frozen span of time engulfed us. If by our presence, touch, and words we could have impacted her recovery, we would have stayed forever. But at one point, a nurse came in and said, "We're going to hook

213

her up to dialyze her, relieve some stress from the kidney. Would you mind waiting outside for a while?" She was followed by a technician who rolled in a metal and plastic cabinet the size of a bar refrigerator—the portable dialysis machine. More dials, buttons and numbers. Their presence focused our concentration on the necessary mechanics of Sylvia's care. Eager for their success, we left them to perform their duties and returned to our usual spot.

John and Angie had joined Cynthia, Michelle and Don in the waiting room. Both John and Angie understood firsthand the serious world of kidney failure, as John had undergone two transplant surgeries. Fortunately, he was doing fine now. They'd both been regular visitors during our surgery in January, offering both of us their support. Now they were here for Maggie.

As John greeted Maggie with a hug, he said, "Don't worry. I went through a lot of this same stuff after my second operation. Geez, for the first six months, it seemed nothing went right. Look at me now. It'll turn out okay, you'll see."

He went over some of the discouraging setbacks after his surgery and convalescence and how he had overcome them. He made it sound as if success after each crisis was inevitable. Such words from an experienced fellow patient were impressive and carried a lot of weight. We began to feel encouraged. Hope resurfaced. Maggie smiled at something Angie said, and I leaned back in my chair to listen to Cynthia and Michelle's chatter. John had restored our faith. We were feeling safe again. The sun had broken through the fog. Our earlier gloom had dissipated. We became a little more animated in our conversation and more comfortable with the waiting.

When it was evident that all there was to do was wait, I considered going through with Don's and my previous plans to go to Sacramento. For several years we'd attended the Sacramento Jazz Festival and had made the usual plans months ago to go this Memorial Day weekend. The previous night, I had thought we'd probably cancel out. But as afternoon approached, it was clear Sylvia would be incommunicado for a couple of days to let the antibiotics work. I thought out loud.

"*Comadre*, what do you think if we go ahead and go to Sacramento after all? Think you'll be okay?"

Without hesitation, she replied, "Go ahead, *comadre*. There's nothing you can do here. Don't worry, I'll be fine. I've got good company here." She slapped Cynthia on the knee and glanced appreciatively at Michelle, John and Angie. "Anyway, I'll probably leave early today myself."

Wavering between guilt and a desire to have a break from the hospital, I hesitated a bit longer. Maggie encouraged me again. "Go on, what can we do to hurry things up? Nothing. You heard Dr. Amend. They're doing all they can. We'll have to trust in that."

As it turned out, we all took her advice. Everyone decided to leave at the same time. Maggie, Cynthia and Michelle were going back to South City, and Don and I headed to Sacramento. I'd left the name of the motel with Cynthia and assured her we'd keep in close touch. Sacramento was just an hour and a half away, so we could be back in that time if needed.

"I'll check in with you later at home, *mija*, to see how things are coming along." I hugged Cynthia goodbye.

That night one of Sylvia's lungs collapsed.

Sunday afternoon, Don and I were back in the ICU waiting room. We'd left Sacramento just as soon as I'd found out about Sylvia's worsening condition. According to Sylvia's nurse, we'd just missed Maggie, Cynthia and my cousin, Maria, by about half an hour. Before entering Sylvia's cubicle, I quizzed the nurse, who sat at her post entering notes into Sylvia's chart. The news was true, but she seemed stable.

When I stepped in to see Sylvia, it chilled my heart. She looked worse than I'd ever seen her before. The facial swelling had increased so that her chin flowed onto her chest, completely obscuring her neck. Her eyes ballooned beneath the stretched lids so that a bit of iris was visible. It was an unnatural sight. Only her nose remained petite, perfectly proportioned despite the invasive tubing. It was incredible that the skin could stretch and swell so much without bursting. Was it possible that additional lines had been added to the previous tangle? It appeared so. I counted eleven hanging bags from three poles, a catheter and a colon tube.

The nurse followed behind me, softly elaborating on Sylvia's condition. "Like I said, it collapsed about one o'clock this morning. She's breathing one hundred percent on the ventilator. Just the one lung collapsed, which is good. But she's getting acidotic, and we're trying to control that." She adjusted the flow of one of the bags, then glanced up at the flashing numbers on the monitor.

"What about the antibiotics?" I asked.

"We're giving her massive doses. I've just increased her…"

The name of the medication was too long, and my brain resisted all the syllables. It was too busy trying to take everything in. The changes were overwhelming, especially in Sylvia's appearance.

"All her doctors have been in—heart, respiratory, Dr. Amend," she went on.

Such information ceased to console me. She was getting worse, and I was going crazy. I stepped near the bed and started to stroke her forehead and speak, when I saw the nurse stiffen as she softly admonished, "We're trying to keep her as quiet as possible. Maybe it would be best if you didn't talk to her right now."

"Oh." I felt like a child who'd been chastised, but promptly obeyed. I stroked her arm, the part above the wrist that was puncture free. Silently I begged her to keep on fighting. All I could do was stare at my poor *mija* and pet her. What a feeling of helplessness. Devoid of thought and afraid to breathe, I felt suspended in time; paralyzed. At the moment, I reasoned that this limbo was the safest place to be.

Eventually, I exited ICU to call home. Cynthia started to cry at the sound of my voice. "I'm so mad at my family. Where are they? Why weren't they there for my *tia* Maggie last night? Only Michelle, Aunt Nen and I were there last night and today. That woman has gone through so much, and no one seems to care." She was angry, tired, and frightened, and I let her vent.

When she paused, I offered what consolation I could. "I know, *mija*. I know. All we can do is what we ourselves wish to do. We can't demand that anyone else follow our lead. Just do what your heart dictates. Don't look around to see who else is there, or you'll go nuts."

After a few moments, her breathing seemed to return to normal. She asked me where I was.

"We got here about four o'clock, just missed you. I've talked to the nurse, and there's nothing new from the time you left. We're going down to the cafeteria for a quick bite, then we'll come back up for a while longer. See you when I get home. Love you." I don't know how consoling that was, but I wasn't feeling particularly inspired. I promised to call her if anything new came up and rang off.

After our cafeteria break, I made another brief visit to ICU. Don patiently read the Sunday newspaper in the waiting room. He hadn't questioned the fact that I wanted to rush back from the Jazz Festival because he knew how important Sylvia was to me. Whatever I needed to do met with his unwavering support. There was never a disapproving word or look. He encouraged me to do what my heart dictated and never complained. That freedom meant a great deal at the time. He felt secure enough not to make me choose between him and my family. I was lucky not to have that additional pressure and appreciated it. He remains my Rock of Gibraltar.

Sylvia's condition remained static. After a half-hour, we left. When I got home, Cynthia and I just hugged. There was nothing new to report, and she knew it without asking. She watched TV in her bedroom and I watched it in the den. I'd given up smoking months prior to the surgery. Never having been a heavy smoker, I did enjoy a couple of cigarettes after dinner at one time. Common sense made me give it up.

Still, whenever I got nervous, I craved a smoke. In the middle of the night, I woke up feeling the need for a cigarette. "To calm my nerves," I lied to myself. I knew Cynthia had a pack in her purse, so I quietly climbed the stairs to her bedroom. Naturally, she was fast asleep. Her purse was next to the nightstand. I tiptoed into her bedroom, bent over the purse and carefully opened it. I spied the shiny cellophane pack and reached in to fish it out. Success. The pack lifted up silently, without clinking keys or other contents. I took it into the adjoining bathroom and quietly extracted two cigarettes. Returning to the bedroom, I placed the cigarettes gently into her bag. Apparently, not gently enough.

"Mom!" She was definitely annoyed at being awakened.

"Sorry, *mija*. I can't sleep."

"Ummpf." She rolled over.

I went back downstairs with my loot and lit up. The first drag sent the tobacco's kick through my system, calming my anxiety attack. It truly is a mental as well as a physical addiction, and while ashamed at giving in to it, I felt a need for it that night. It was just past midnight, and the only thing on TV was reruns. I watched *I Love Lucy*. Lighting up one cigarette, I smoked through the episode, staring at the familiar faces, not thinking, not feeling, just staring and smoking. Soon both cigarettes were ashes. By this time, it was after two. I didn't have to work the following day since it was Memorial Day, so I stayed up a bit longer. Finally, unable to keep my eyes open, I went to bed, hoping not to think or dream. My real nightmare would catch me awake.

20

Let This Cup Pass

Monday and Tuesday brought no change despite the aggressive antibiotic cocktail treatment. Wednesday, I took half a vacation day because my mind was jailed in ICU and I simply couldn't concentrate on anything else. John continued to be understanding. As long as I went in to handle the morning mail and take care of anything urgent, taking the afternoon off wasn't a problem.

As part of our regular routine, I dropped Maggie off at the hospital on my way to work in the morning. Later, when I arrived at the hospital, Michelle would have brought her aunt some lunch, and they'd be sitting together in the waiting room. Michelle usually stayed with her until I showed up.

"Hi!" I said to my *comadre*. "Oh, good, you've eaten." I walked straight to Michelle and gave her an appreciative hug. "You take good care of your *tia, mija*."

Maggie half-smiled and nodded. "Yes, she sure does."

Scooting the green naugahyde ottoman in front of Maggie and Michelle, I sat down and asked, "Well... anything new?"

"Not yet, still the same." Maggie sighed. "Come in with me, *comadre*. You talk to the nurse. I get confused, and I'm not sure if I'm getting everything she says."

Michelle turned to me. "I'm going back down to my office, *tia*. See you after five. Will you still be here? Can I have a ride home?"

219

"Sure, *mija*," I replied. "We'll probably be here at least until six. So take your time. We won't leave without you."

Michelle explained, "My supervisor has been pretty good about my coming up here, but I do need to get some work done. Since you'll be here 'til six, I'll work a little overtime. See you then." She walked toward the elevator and disappeared.

Maggie and I gravitated toward the double doors that pulled us into another world.

She can't swell up much more, I thought. This was not my Sylvia lying there. Forgetting I wasn't supposed to, I spoke to my godchild. "Hi, *mija*. Can you feel the antibiotics working? You letting them do their job?"

The nurse looked in and announced, "Dr. Amend talked to Dr. Adams, the heart specialist. They're watching her very carefully. So is the respiratory doctor. She's got lots of people watching over her." Undoubtedly, these words were meant to comfort. But we were both becoming immune to comforting words and unable to draw much relief from them.

One of the IVs tolled, and the nurse adjusted its regulator. She walked around and checked several of the other bags, looked up at the monitor, returned to her podium and filled in little boxes with numbers. Always lots of numbers.

As she intently scrawled into the day's journal, two men in white coats came in and stopped to speak to her. Apparently she was updating the doctors who were part of Sylvia's medical team. They listened somberly, nodded occasionally. Finally, they walked into the cubicle, stopping by the ventilator. They were the respiratory team. The three continued their discussion. We kept silent. After a few minutes of looking at the graphs and taking readings, one of the doctors turned as if to exit the room.

I anxiously asked, "When you're through with your examination, doctor, could you please talk to us?"

"Certainly." He stepped over to check something in the nurse's chart. They whispered. She reported, he listened. He commented, she elaborated. He ordered, she wrote hurriedly. We continued waiting, praying that our silence enabled them to concentrate on the business of healing. The second doctor left the breathing machine after checking it and joined the others at the podium. More whispering. The first doctor came and stood beside us with the same immobile expression that he'd worn since arriving.

"She's not responding to the antibiotics," he began bluntly. "Both lungs have collapsed. Additionally, there's not one spot on either lung that's not diseased. The ventilator is doing all her breathing for her."

That such catastrophic, hideous words can be uttered without screaming, without rage, or without passion must be a critical part of doctors' training. The cold logic of his assessment, the experience and expertise with which he gave us his evaluation, staggered my senses. I didn't see Maggie's reaction, but knew that her senses had been similarly assaulted.

"Both lungs?" I heard myself repeat unbelievingly.

He nodded.

"But a couple of days ago she was doing thirty per cent of her own breathing. Why isn't she getting better with all the antibiotics?"

"I don't know," he admitted.

I wanted to scream. "Why don't you know!"

How dare the gods in white jackets not be infallible! As much as I wished to denounce him as a liar, there was no escaping his candor. But I greatly resented how he sounded so dogmatic. Some of my hostility must have surfaced, because he stepped backwards.

"Maybe the antibiotics haven't kicked in yet," he said quietly. "Let's hope they do soon. We're doing all we can." He raised his brows and pursed his lips with a "That's all I can say for now" look. In all fairness, it could have been an effort to show some empathy. If it was, it fell short. We didn't know how to respond. He used our silence to slip away.

I replayed his words over and over in my head. Not one spot on either lung was free of disease? When had the second lung collapsed? Where on earth were those damned antibiotics? Why in hell weren't they working!

"Dear God, is it miracle time, or are you reclaiming her?" These thoughts immobilized me. Had we gone through so much together for this? The possibility of losing her had probably been subconsciously buried inside me since before our surgery. But once we'd recuperated, I'd acknowledged our success, dispelled my fears and reveled in the fact that we'd made it. I had thought we were out of the woods five months ago. We certainly had never anticipated losing her to lung disease or any other non-kidney-related ailment. What bitter irony. It was shattering. All I could think of was, "Please let this cup pass, Lord."

I couldn't guess what thoughts raced through Maggie, what profound anguish pressed against her heart. We sat, numbed into silence, beside a peacefully still Sylvia. We stood for an indeterminable length of time. I can't remember when we returned to the waiting room or if we had dinner. We left the hospital less hopeful that night, unhinged by the reality of what might lay ahead.

On Thursday, June first, I took another half day's vacation. Again, I found Michelle chaperoning her *tía* in the sun-soaked waiting room. She rose when I arrived, and we shared a warm embrace. She was too sad to say anything. Without greeting me, Maggie stood up quickly and said, "Come on, *comadre*, I haven't been in for a while." She looked so drained. Not waiting for a reply, she led Michelle and me into ICU, reminding me of a quail with her brood.

I took a chair only at Maggie's insistence. I hardly looked at Sylvia because I couldn't take my eyes off the monitors. Oxygenation level was in the high eighties to low nineties, which was not bad. Blood pressure numbers were improved, but not great. Pulse rate was close to normal. Scanning the more positive numbers, my heart beat faster.

"*Comadre*, I think the numbers are better than yesterday. What do you think?" Mustn't sound too buoyant.

"Yes, I think so, too." Maggie had a way of nodding vigorously when she was in total agreement, and she was doing that now.

The nurse entered. "We're going to change one of the lines now. You'll have to step out for a moment."

As she entered, a group of white coats came into ICU, blocking our exit. Dr. Amend was in their midst, along with the heart specialist and a female doctor we hadn't seen before. They huddled behind our nurse's stand, sharing information. The nurse, in the meantime, had proceeded to work on one of Sylvia's lines in spite of the fact that we were still in the cubicle. We were waiting for the doctors' group to disperse so we could move toward the exit. I kept looking at the monitor, so much so that one of the passing nurses kindly suggested that I not contract what they called "monitor fixation."

"Remember, now. It's part of the overall picture, not the entire picture. Try not to concentrate on them so much." She said it as kindly as she knew how, and I appreciated it, but I couldn't seem to take her advice. I noticed a drop in the blood pressure numbers and was mentally puzzling over them when I noted our nurse doing the same thing. She slipped over to the group of doctors and calmly directed their attention to Sylvia's monitor. Almost in unison, they lunged toward our cubicle, eyeing the monitor and surrounding the bed.

One of them ordered, "Please wait outside. We'll call you back as soon as we can."

We sat at the familiar round table in the corner of the waiting room rather than on the sofa we were so tired of. Anxiety, curiosity and fear enveloped us. For a while, we remained silent. Minutes passed. Gradually, we began talking again.

"Did Rolando get over his ear infection?" I asked my *comadre*.

"Yes, but the doctor doesn't want to put tubes in. You know Sylvia and Gilbert had the same thing when they were little. Remember? I know all about it, but no, he doesn't want to put them in. Don't know what he's waiting for. He's going to have them sometime, anyway." She was quite indignant that her grandson couldn't have the ear drainage tubes she thought were required. We talked about domestic matters, swapped family tidbits, complained about our aches and pains, and even commented on the progress of the O.J. Simpson trial. A comforting normalcy settled in.

About forty minutes later, Dr. Amend joined us. He pulled up a chair, placed both arms on the table, clasped his hands and said, "We just pulled her out of a sudden drop in blood pressure. She's okay, though." He touched Maggie's hand with a comforting tap. "But she's still a very sick girl." He paused. "We've all just had a discussion about this—the heart and lung doctors, everyone. We need to talk about it." Switching his gaze from Maggie to me and back to Maggie, he took a deep breath and said, "If this should happen again, we're not going to interfere or use any electricity."

I blinked. My lips felt cemented shut. Had I heard correctly? Maggie caught her breath. I stared at Dr. Amend. I must have heard wrong. He was looking back at us, eyes full of compassion and too much candor.

Slowly my mouth began to work. "What are you saying?"

With deliberate patience, he elaborated. "She's not getting better. We don't know why the antibiotics aren't working, but they're not." Frustration tinged his words. "They should have kicked in by now. The only thing keeping her alive is the ventilator. If she has another drop in pressure like this last one, we've decided not to use any electricity to keep her going."

I was dumbfounded. Mute. Turning to Maggie, I realized she had understood what I desperately sought to reject.

"The antibiotics might still kick in, we don't know," Dr. Amend said. "We're doing everything we can think of, Maggie. She's got more specialists than I can count." It was obviously painful for him to report on the findings of his colleagues, but his pain couldn't soften our shock or heartache.

Those Madonna-like eyes of my *comadre* teared up. She whispered, "I know, Dr. Amend, I know you're doing all you can. Don't blame yourself, you've done your best. You and Dr. Vicente…" She stopped in mid-sentence, turned her face towards the door, stood and walked out as if she had heard the calling of some mythical siren, luring her to some secret rendezvous impossible to resist. She moved as if bewitched toward the siren's song, heeding its call as she passed through those double doors.

I sat frozen in front of the man who'd always helped Sylvia, who was in charge of making her better and who'd successfully done that several times before. How many times had he plucked her out of danger and brought her back to safety? What had gone wrong this time?

His words crushed me, robbing me of breath. I lacked the energy, will or presence of mind to respond. Everything was so confusing. My throat thickened. Finally, I heard my own voice. "I thought I'd given her a magic bullet last January. I thought she'd get BETTER. I thought she was going to LIVE!"

I was crying my tearless cry. I covered my face, sobbing my heart out into my hands. In the background, Dr. Amend hastened to comfort me. His words slammed against an erected barrier. Though I heard his voice, his words were meaningless. I'd never believe in him again. I heard the chair scrape against the vinyl floor as he left. A soft sobbing made me realize that Michelle was nearby. I went and sat next to her, placing my arm around her shoulders. Neither of us spoke.

The family living between my *compadres'* South City house and the house of my former in-laws was the Huerta family. They were from the same small Mexican town the Zertuches were from. Both my *compadres* and my ex-husband and I had baptized one of their boys. Maggie and Mando had baptized the middle son, Hector, and Lupe and I had baptized the younger son, Eduardo. We treated each other as family, participating in each other's parties, celebrations, good times and bad times. Terri, Sylvia and Gilbert had grown up and played with the Huerta children. The boys had always treated the girls as sisters and Gil as another brother. They were now in their late twenties or early thirties. Because of the families' closeness, it wasn't surprising to see two of them, Armandito and Hector, walk in on Michelle and me as we attempted to console one another. In fact, nothing could have been more natural. Their arrival was comforting.

Hector, about twenty-six years old, slid into the chair recently vacated by Dr. Amend. His handsome features were sharpened by concern. The blue-black hair, always trimmed to perfection, was cropped close. He always had that crisply-fresh look, even in work clothes after a full day on the job. Instincts alerted, he asked, "Where's my *nina?*" He meant Maggie.

Maggie was Hector's godmother, and they shared the same bond that linked Sylvia and me. This was another reason his presence seemed so natural and fitting. His older brother, Armandito (always known by the diminutive version of his name, Armando), stood opposite me. He'd been named after Mando because Armandito's dad and Mando were such close friends. With arms folded against his chest, he waited for some kind of reply. Our reticence seemed to make him wary.

"She's in with Sylvia. Dr. Amend just left," I said. "It's not good. Really not good. If she has another crisis, they're not going to save her by any artificial means. They're going to keep medicating her, but they'll let nature take its course if…" I couldn't finish.

Hector's dark eyes filled with tears. Armandito tightened his lips until they became rimmed in white.

"Let's go in. I need to see her." I grabbed my shoulder bag and led them through the doors. They followed in silence. Michelle stayed behind.

"Can we all come in?" I asked the nurse.

"Sure. If you'll just stand against the wall so I can have access to the left side of the bed, it'll be fine. Need another chair?"

Two chairs were already pushed against the wall. "No thank you."

Maggie was standing on the right side of the bed, holding Sylvia's hand in hers and saying, "Come on, Chiva. Get better, *mija*, you can do it. Don't be so stubborn. Always, you're so stubborn." The cadence of her softly-accented English was like a spoken lullabye.

Without saying anything, Armandito and Hector sat in the chairs, absorbing the mood and fears of the situation. Sylvia's appearance must have staggered them. I stood at the foot of the bed, silent, still stunned by the reality of her condition and the sentence Dr. Amend had given.

Suddenly, Hector popped up, took Maggie's hand in his, turned to his brother, urging him up from his chair, and reached out for his hand. With his eyes on me, he urged Armandito to take my hand. Armandito obeyed. We clung to one another with one hand, our free hands resting on Sylvia.

"You've heard of hands on?" Hector said with authority. "Well, that's what we're going to do. We're going to give her our strength and energy and let it pass through us to her."

We gratefully accepted his command. It was as if we simultaneously thought, "Oh, of course, this will work. Why didn't we think of it before?"

We stood linked, gazing at Sylvia, our love emanating over her, bathing her still form. We were resolute that she must be healed. We were determined to will her to health. Someone started the Our Father, and we all joined in. Minutes passed. Our infusion had no outward sign of success, but we were not discouraged. In fact, the effect was uplifting. If only Sylvia could hear Armandito and Hector.

Shortly afterward, the day nurse was approached by her evening replacement, and we were asked to leave for a while. Apparently, there'd be no eavesdropping on today's report. As we sat in our familiar spots in the waiting room, the sun streamed shamelessly through the wall of windows. We received no solace from it, even though it filled the room with warmth and sunbeams. It seemed cruel that the day should be so sunny.

My Joe walked in about six o'clock to find us talking in short spurts. He joined our circle, and he and the Huerta boys exchanged warm greetings. His *tia* Maggie got the usual bear hug, as did Michelle and me. I could tell that Maggie was greatly touched by all the boys' presence. Their love for her and Sylvia was so evident, one couldn't help but be comforted by it. Joe's reaction when we filled him in on Sylvia's condition was silent comprehension and an occasional nod. At the end of our accounting, he leaned back in his chair, turned his head towards his *tia* and, touching her hand, said, "It'll be all right, *tia*. It has to be all right."

She gave him a weak smile, then worried out loud, "I think I should call Terri, *comadre*, and have her and Gilbert come down right away. They can leave Rolando with my sister. Oh, I hope she can come. She says she doesn't want to, but I don't know if she means it."

"Don't worry, *comadre*. She'll come," I said.

I was confident saying this because I knew Cynthia and Terri had talked on the phone the previous evening. Terri admitted to Cynthia that she'd resisted going to the hospital because she didn't want to see her sister so ill. The possibilities frightened her.

"I just don't think I could handle it." Terri had cried over the phone.

Cynthia scolded her. "Right, and I can? None of us can! Look, your mom needs you. She needs to have her children around her. You've got to come down. Don't go in and see Sylvia if you don't want to, but be there for your mom. She just needs you to be there, that's all."

I'm sure more passed between them that wasn't shared with me. But I felt comfortable enough to encourage Maggie to call Terri.

In reality, Terri had always been there for Maggie. After all, it was she who had given Sylvia her first kidney donation. When her father died in 1985, she was only twenty-three. Yet she became the stalwart supporter of her mother through the turmoil of finding a new home and starting a new life in a different city. She and Sylvia had shared many difficult times during those first years of Maggie's widowhood and their loss of a father. Through it all, they'd always been there for their mom. Later, when Sylvia had repeated setbacks due to her kidney problem, it was Terri whom Maggie relied on for moral support.

There was never any doubt that Terri had always been there for Maggie, and now was no exception. But there comes a saturation point where it doesn't seem possible to absorb any more of what life deals out. Perhaps now was this time for Terri. On the other hand, she may have felt a premonition that this was the climax of Sylvia's battle, and the possibility terrified her. In her fear, Terri might have clung to her refuge at home. Who could blame her? In the end, I knew she'd be there simply because she'd always been there. No one could have received as much from a sister as Sylvia had from hers.

Maggie wore a contented smile when she returned from making her call. "Terri said she's already called Gilbert, and they're driving down as soon as they can. She'll leave the baby with my sister. They'll both be here sometime during the night." Relieved, Maggie repeated, "Yes, they're coming."

The Huertas eventually left. Joe and I tried to talk Maggie into joining us for dinner in the cafeteria. No luck. We took the elevator down to the cafeteria, and as the doors opened, Dr. Juliet Melzer, my surgeon, walked in.

"What are you doing here?" she asked.

"Sylvia's in ICU. It's not looking too good at the moment, I'm afraid."

While I hoped for words of encouragement, she merely said, "Oh, yes. Dr. Amend told me." There was a pause. "She's a very sick girl." Her eyes were sad as they looked directly into mine. She said nothing else. At the time, I felt she'd been insensitive. Surely, she could have offered some words of encouragement, extended a little hope, shown some sympathy. In looking back, I realize that it would have been unprofessional for her to do so. We finished the elevator ride in silence.

The chance encounter with Dr. Melzer had a sobering effect that caused a horrific weight to compress my heart. Could it really be true, then? Could it be possible that Sylvia would really die? She who'd vanquished so many other threats? My brave, spirited, lively *mija*? I told myself not to think this way. Stop this nonsense. It couldn't be; wouldn't be. I sought to quell the panic welling up inside me. Exiting the elevator, I followed Joe to the cafeteria line.

We each grabbed what we wanted. As hospital cafeterias went, it wasn't bad. There were choices to please fat-intake watchers, anti-carb dieters, pizza fans, Mexican food aficionados, sandwich customers, salad freaks and dessert lovers. I think Joe got a sandwich. I picked at a salad and sipped water. Since neither of us are ever at a loss for words when we're together, our conversation was animated. For a while, we ignored the topic most on our minds. Eventually he asked, "So, who's been here?"

"Your *tio* Serjio and *tia* Josie, Nen and Charlie, Concha and Ramon" (the Huerta parents), "Concha's sister, Noni, your grandpa and Uncle Henry, Angie and John, and, of course, Hector and Armandito. Cynthia was here over the weekend, and she'll be here later. Oh, and Michelle has been here watching over your *tia* as often as her job allows. She gets Maggie to eat, which is big."

"Think I should take tomorrow off?" His nonchalant delivery didn't belie his concern.

"Ummm, let's wait and see what happens. I keep waiting for those damned antibiotics to kick in. For God's sake, the nurse says they're giving her cocktails with mega doses of antibiotics, three different ones. I don't know why…" I sipped from my glass to quiet myself.

We ended up talking about his work, a pending business trip to Oregon, and my own work. I vividly remember laughing towards the end of our twenty-minute break, but not why or about what.

Afterwards, we returned to the ninth floor. As we approached the waiting room, we heard different voices. At the door, Sylvia's best friend, Elisa, and her husband, Jim, met us. They'd been talking with her cousin Angie, who'd arrived while Joe and I were downstairs. By now, Cynthia was also in the room with her *tia*, Michelle, her grandfather, and her uncles, Henry and Charlie. As inappropriate as it may sound, taking into consideration why we were all there, there was a cheerful, consoling solace from the familial chatter. A laugh erupted from Maggie as she teased one of her nephews. Charlie and Joe exchanged their knowledge of the latest redneck jokes, the current craze in humor. Cynthia, Michelle, Elisa and Angie were engrossed in conversation, and I caught up on family affairs with my ex-in laws, with whom I still enjoyed a mutually affectionate relationship.

As ten o'clock neared, Charlie turned to his sister-in-law, Maggie. "I'm going back in for a minute to say goodnight. Then I've got to go; early meeting in the morning." Charlie and my cousin Nen faced a forty-five-minute drive back home to San Carlos.

"I'll go in with you," Maggie said.

Cynthia took advantage of Maggie's absence to slip out to the public telephone in the hallway to call Stockton. Cell phones weren't the rage then. When Terri answered, she listened for a moment before responding. "No, Terri. It's serious, really serious, not like before. She's not doing good. They've told us outright they're not going to do anything to save her if she has another crisis like this afternoon's. There's no improvement. No response to the medicine…"

Elisa, who could overhear the phone conversation, jumped up from her chair and ran toward the double doors, stopping just in front of them. "It's not true!" she cried. "She is going to get better. She can't die!" She froze in place, not knowing which direction was safest. Denial babbled from her as her husband rose to enfold her in her arms. Offering his wife a tissue, he led her back to a chair, where she sat sobbing into her hands.

Cynthia bent her ear into the phone to hear what Terri was saying. Then she hung up and returned to a waiting audience anxious to know what had been said.

"She's just waiting for Gilbert to get there. Should be there any minute, then they'll be on their way. She's crying, Mom, but she had to know the truth."

"You did right, *mija*. Thank you."

Cynthia sat down next to me as Maggie exited the ICU with Charlie and Nen. They said their goodbyes and left while Maggie came back to us. "I hope they're coming," she said, her thoughts turned inward. We knew who "they" were. I nodded toward Cynthia, indicating she had some news.

"Yes, they are, *tia*. Gilbert is due there any minute. That's all Terri's waiting for. Guess he had to work late. They should be leaving soon."

Suddenly, we were all quiet and visibly weary. Most of the family had trickled out. Joe left, giving me his girlfriend's phone number in case I needed to call him during the night. I knew he didn't want to be alone. Lisa shared his deepest emotions, and I was thankful he was going to be with her.

Just before midnight, Cynthia announced that she couldn't wait any longer for her cousins to arrive from Stockton because she had to get up early for work. Saying her goodbyes, she left with the usual, "Call me, Mom, if anything happens."

Maggie, Michelle and I went in to see Sylvia. As we kept vigil near the bedside, we were each absorbed in our own thoughts. A blessed mental numbness overtook me, and I was able to gaze and touch without feeling pain. The nurse flitted in and out. We had no further questions of her. I shifted my feet and looked over at Maggie, who was standing directly across from me on the opposite side of the bed. I heard myself break the silence.

"I've never thanked you for giving her to me to baptize, *comadre*. From that day, she's always been so very special to me. Thank you so much." A sob stuck in my throat. Flashbacks of every stage in Sylvia's life reeled through my mind. I clearly saw a toddler's chubby face, the grammar school tomboy, the awkward youngster, the blossoming teenager, the *quinceañera* deb, our water-skier, those cool dance moves, and her graduation photo, my favorite picture. The last vision I had of her was the one I still remember as if it were yesterday. That of Sylvia's face lifted up to receive the rain as we walked.

"No, thank YOU," my *comadre* whispered back. "You were always very special to her, too. You were so much alike in your thinking." She mimicked Sylvia, "That's my *nina*. Don't you say anything about her."

We managed a smile before the weight of what was happening again closed in. I excused myself to go to the restroom. Both Maggie and Michelle nodded without shifting their gaze from the bed. It was almost one o'clock on Friday morning. As I went down the hall, I looked out the windows. The darkness outside offered a timelessness, a darkness that could hold back the dawn. Here in the hospital we seemed cocooned in the now. It held us in its embrace, offering no progression, no loss. The dual worlds inside and outside the hospital were hushed. If only time would remain still and tranquil. I wanted so much to be suspended in its dimension, its solace. I said a silent prayer. "Let this cup pass, Lord." But I couldn't bring myself to think about the second half: "Thy will be done."

21

Vigil of Hope

When I re-entered Sylvia's cubicle, Terri and Gilbert were there. An unbroken stream of tears poured down Terri's blushed cheeks as she murmured her sister's nickname. "Chiva, Chiva." She repeated it over and over in a plaintive chant, perhaps realizing she was using that term of endearment for the last time.

Gilbert stood next to his mother in silence, his arms about her shoulders, jaws clenched shut, his eyes staring at his sister in her induced slumber. I wondered what impact her physical condition was having on him since he hadn't seen her for a couple of weeks. His face held a restrained anguish.

As usual, my eyes wandered and locked on the monitor's flashing numbers. Gently elbowing Maggie on the arm, I gestured with my chin towards the box. The nurse was at her post, writing, always writing. Shortly, she got down from the stool and entered the cubicle to perform some task. Guardedly, I called her attention to the monitor.

"Looks like her blood pressure is up."

With the exception of shifting her eyes upward for a cursory glance, the nurse's expression registered no change. She simply uttered, "Hmm."

"Isn't that a good sign?" I begged for a bit of encouragement.

"That part's slightly better, but she's still very acidotic."

Not a smidgen of hope from that quarter, although she did offer some enlightenment. I listened carefully while she explained that the body's chemistry changes when the vital organs aren't functioning normally. The RH factors become unbalanced, and the blood becomes acidic, which can be dangerous because it causes a terrific strain on the heart. In short, being acidotic is not a good thing.

The weight of the nurse's discouraging response, coupled with the lateness of the hour, began to wear us down. I looked toward Maggie, from whom I'd take my lead. Terri and Gilbert's presence had definitely comforted her. Some of the anxiety had left her face. "Let's go," she sighed. "We'll be back in a few hours."

To Sylvia she said, "*Mija*, hold tight. Rest, let the medicines do their work. We'll be back soon." She planted a tender kiss on her forehead.

We each gave her a kiss and said we'd be back. I took a last glance at the monitor and thought out loud. "I think she knows that Terri and Gilbert are here. Look, her blood pressure is coming up."

Maggie gave a nod, wishing my words to be true.

As we passed the nurse's station, the nurse said, "Oh, I'm glad you're going home. Get some rest. If you want to call at any time, here's another one of my cards. Feel free to call. Let's see. I've got your numbers in case the doctor wants to call you?" She flipped a few pages, then said, "Yes, they're here."

I checked to make sure my home and office numbers were correct. The last time I'd checked the clock, it was about two-thirty in the morning.

Gilbert left in his car to meet Terri and me at my townhouse. Maggie, Michelle, Terri and I went in my car. I dropped Maggie off with Michelle, who lived very close to the hospital. She was planning to return to ICU at eight o'clock in the morning when Michelle left for work. Terri and I proceeded to San Bruno.

Five minutes after we arrived at my place, Gilbert knocked at the front door. "Where's Cindy?" he asked.

"Asleep, she has to go to work in the morning," I answered. "Come on, let's have something to eat and drink."

For the first time in our lives, I offered my niece and nephew a drink. They were well over twenty-one, and I figured if they were mature enough to handle the current situation, they could handle a little nightcap.

"I've got some rum, vodka, whiskey, beer, tequila?"

"I'll take a tequila, *tia*," Terri said.

"Make mine beer," Gilbert said as he slid onto one of the dining room chairs.

Our snack consisted of microwaved frozen burritos whose benefit lay in being warm sustenance rather than gourmet treats. Before joining them at the table, I made myself a scalding cup of Ovaltine and poured a jigger of Frangelico into it. We talked softly about their commute from Stockton, their impressions of Sylvia's condition, and the doctors' prognoses until the subjects were as exhausted as we were. I was the first to excuse myself.

"*Mijo*, I've made up the couch downstairs for you. Terri, you can either sleep with Cynthia or me. You know where everything is if you need towels or anything. I'm off to bed."

"Okay, *gracias, tia*."

"Don't stay up too late. We've got an early start in the morning. What do you think about getting up at…" I looked at the clock on the microwave. "Geez, four o'clock! Umm, how about around nine?"

"I'm going whenever I wake up," Gilbert said.

Terri instructed him, "Wake me when you get up if I'm not up yet."

"Me, too, Gil. Don't leave without me," I told him. "Terri, if you don't go up with Gil, you can go with me, so don't worry."

I left the pair at the dining room table, where I'm sure they had private matters to discuss. When I set the alarm on my bedstand clock, it was just past four. I was asleep in seconds.

The clanging of the telephone, so natural sounding in daylight, always registers such shock when it awakens me at night. When I answer it at such times, I'm not thinking straight, but my mouth goes on anyway.

"Who? Yes, it is." I sat up, half annoyed and wholly confused. The voice belonged to one of the UCSF staff doctors we'd met earlier during routine hospital rounds. She spoke gently, calmly, so matter-of-factly, so terribly civilized.

"What!" I shouted.

She repeated her statement, "I'm afraid Sylvia's heart gave out. She died at four-ten. It was sudden and very peaceful, if that's any consolation. I'm so sorry."

"But we just left her!" I shouted.

This was totally insane. Was I dreaming? How could she have possibly died? And without us there? It couldn't be. We hadn't considered her as being on her deathbed; she was just very ill. My level of denial was so profound that I couldn't accept her words. I felt gutted. When I'd seen the improved numbers on the monitor just before leaving the hospital, I'd been so hopeful. I was convinced it was the beginning of a turnaround for her.

When it finally registered that I wasn't being lied to and should respond, I managed, "Oh... I... We'll be right there."

Before both my feet were on the carpet, Terri poked her head through the bedroom door, and I could hear Gil's deep voice behind her.

"What is it, *tia?* Who was that?"

My arms flew towards her in a wild embrace. "She died, *mija.* At four-ten, her heart gave out. That was the lady doctor." Oddly, I wasn't crying. The shock was too overwhelming.

Terri gave out a short wail. "No! Oh, God, no."

Her sobs snapped me back. I released her as she fell onto the bed crying. I threw off my nightgown and began searching for jeans, anything, to cover up and rush out. My paralysis changed to a frenzied panic, a need to do something. Anything.

Sobs bounced off the short, narrow hallway between the bathroom and the den, where Gil's couch-bed was barely rumpled. I heard him moan and knew he'd heard. Soon the three of us were scurrying around. In our distress, we grabbed the clothes we'd just discarded minutes ago and struggled to get them on. Terri was in the upstairs bathroom, dressing and crying. I bounded up to Cynthia's room, still disbelieving—knowing that when we arrived at the hospital, we'd learn it was all a mistake.

As I reached the foot of her bed, she rolled over. "Yeah?" A long pause followed.

I stood motionless, the words sticking in my throat.

"What?" she asked again.

I finally whispered, "She's gone, *mija*. They just called."

The eyes were distorted with pain as she covered them, turned her head and crushed her face into the pillow to sob. I touched her briefly, not wanting to lose time. "We're on our way."

As I flew out of the room, I heard her say, "I can't go. I need to be at work early. Tsk…" She was definitely torn.

I went back, stood in the doorway and said, "I know, *mija*. I know. Don't worry. The important thing is that you were there for her when it counted. You did all you could." Those words held heartfelt conviction. I added, "I'll call you later."

Suddenly, I remembered something important, sped back downstairs to the kitchen phone and hurriedly punched some numbers.

"Michelle? *Mija*, have you heard from the hospital?"

"No, *tia*." A slight hesitation was followed by, "Is she gone?"

"Yes, they just called. Her heart gave out about four-ten."

I could hear her soft voice repeating the words to her *tia*. Sounds of movement carried through the phone. No moans—simply determined motions.

Remembering I was in a hurry, I said, "We're leaving now. Want me to pick you up?"

She asked Maggie, then responded, "Yes, please."

I felt so terribly inept. How sterile and matter-of-fact the notification had been. Even as I uttered the words, I hated how briefly this tragedy was expressed. No words can capture death.

There was nothing left to say except, "See you in about twenty minutes."

One more call.

"*Mijo?*"

"Yeah, Mom?"

"I'm afraid she's gone. Died about four-ten. We're on our way up there now."

A deep, heavy sigh flowed through the line. "Thanks for calling. I'll call you later, Mom, if I don't go up. Drive careful."

Just one more to go. Hurry.

"Charlie? The hospital just called. She died about four-ten."

"Oh, my God."

"Will you please call Serjio and everyone else? We're on our way up to the hospital again."

"Sure, take care. Call me later, lady."

Charlie often called me "lady," and the familiarity of it always made me feel like he was a real brother and not just a brother-in-law. I knew I could depend on him to let everyone know.

I lunged back downstairs, one arm pushing through my sweater and the other grabbing for my purse. Gil was walking out the front door in long, measured steps.

"See you there," he called over his shoulder.

I yelled upstairs. "*Mija*, will you please call the girls before you go to work?" The term "girls" meant my sisters. To my surprise, Cynthia was flying down the stairs, Terri close behind. Both were in my face before I'd finished the sentence.

"I'm going with you."

22

At the End of the Corridor

The hospital hallway led us on. It was probably close to five o'clock in the morning. Dawn had not yet broken, adding to the bleak darkness in our hearts. Finally, the corridor ended, and here we were facing the familiar double doors marked ICU. The six of us, Maggie, Terri, Gil, Cynthia, Michelle and I, paused. It was an eternal moment, crammed with a hope that might dissolve if we dared to move. But once Maggie pushed forward, we stirred to follow.

The night nurse, whom we'd last seen about one-thirty in the morning, stood outside Sylvia's cubicle. At the swooshing of the door, she turned and walked toward Maggie with outstretched arms.

"I'm so sorry. She went very peacefully, if that's any consolation."

Maggie nodded. "Thank you. Thank you all for your help." She returned the hug before breaking loose to float toward Sylvia's bed. I followed my *comadre*, moving to the opposite side of the bed. It was true; she was gone. The inconceivable had become fact. Touching Sylvia's thigh underneath the cold sheet, I dropped to my knees, burying my face into the thin coverlet to wail uncontrollably.

"Chiva, Chiva. *Mija.* You were supposed to get better. Why, *mija,* why didn't you?" I heard myself crying as I'd never cried. The anguish drowned out all else, and I was aware of nothing except the empty shell that had once housed her spirit. It had failed her, and us.

For thirty years, eleven months and one week, she'd been ours, and in that time, neither Maggie nor I had expected to relinquish her essence before the end of our own lives. Sylvia, our gift, our daughter, my god-child, gone from this earth.

At some point, I became aware of Cynthia's hand on my shoulder and the comfort her touch sought to give. Its presence made me stop crying to look up. Tears streamed down her face. The Sylvia she'd loved was as precious to her as her own sister would have been if she'd had one. Nothing in her twenty-six years had prepared her for such grief. I've never been at such a loss to comfort my own child. With her tender touch, she made me feel more like the child than the parent.

I glanced over at Maggie. Again, she took on the aspect of the Madonna as depicted in the *Pieta*. She was a study in quiet, sorrowful resignation as she gently stroked her daughter's hair back from her forehead. Emptied of tears, she tenderly repeated words of farewell, assuring Sylvia that all her suffering was over, and now, as she joined her father, she knew their reunion would be a joyous one. Her acceptance of Sylvia's death revealed the resolve of an unfaltering faith.

We encircled our newly-initiated angel. Terri and Gilbert flanked their mother. Michelle, eyes red from crying, was part of the grieving circle. She stood in silence next to her favorite *tia*. Ultimately, the sense of serenity that Maggie generated soothed us all.

As I looked at Sylvia's face, I noticed that her eyes, though screened by smooth, creamy lids, looked peaceful and not as swollen. Her features reflected a tranquility absent during her struggle of the past week. She was so peaceful. Her ultimate destination had been reached, and I drew consolation from that.

Yet inwardly I was still conflicted. I kept thinking, "How can I leave you here? Dear God, I can't leave her." She looked so serene lying there. I just wanted to gaze at her. And I detested the thought of walking out into a world that didn't include her. I continued to marvel at my *comadre*, who bore her loss with such quiet grace. I yearned to absorb some of it.

We were silent, paralyzed in the knowledge that we had to accept this dreadful reality. I could only draw solace from the fact that she was in heaven with Mando. For this I was glad.

I don't know how long we lingered beside her bed. It was Maggie who closed the curtain on our long vigil. When she chose the moment to leave, we accepted and followed.

We buried our Sylvia on June 5, 1995, at Holy Cross Cemetery in Colma, across from her dad and not too far from where her grand-parents would eventually rest. In the manner of our faith and Mexican culture, many relatives and friends accompanied us for the wake, the rosary and the funeral Mass.

Being showered with the comfort of such tremendous support and condolences means much to us in times of grief. It reinforces the alliance between family and friends and strengthens our commitment to one another. Communal recognition of our brief time here on earth is an effective mortar for cementing these bonds. To have so many people pause from their daily routines is a real tribute to the deceased.

Sylvia's life was celebrated by hundreds. Many were young adults. Aside from her cousins, there were camping and water skiing friends, school pals, the children of family friends, and other old friends who came to pay their respects. Because Sylvia loved seeing guys in jeans, the pall bearers, all relatives, had decided to wear jeans with sports coats and ties. It was a final tribute to their fun-loving Sylvia. One high school friend who knew of Sylvia's love of riding motorcycles snuck a miniature toy cycle into her casket before it was sealed shut. She summoned many other loving remembrances. Each one, regardless of how small, touched us deeply.

Days after the funeral, after Maggie, Terri and Gil had returned to Stockton, Terri and Cynthia resumed their long-distance telephone con-versations. Terri, a poetic soul, searched tirelessly for the right words to place on Sylvia's headstone, sharing her compositions with Cynthia over the phone. I heard some of her poems, and they were heartfelt and lengthy, trying to capture so much. I couldn't help commenting to Cynthia, "*Mija*, I wonder if Terri is aware that they charge you by the letter on the headstones. This is going to run into a lot of money."

Cynthia relayed this information to Terri the next time they spoke. In the meantime, I'd jotted down a few shortened phrases taken from Terri's words and mixed in some of my thoughts, and we came up with "Angel, Watch Over Us." While Terri had drafted many lines of creative prose in her young lifetime, the practicality and suitability of the chosen phrase made it, in my opinion, the right one. I dare to think that our Sylvia might be pleased with it. With the wording for the headstone chosen, a finality seemed to drop into place. The reality of resuming daily life faced us all.

It took months before my sorrow dissipated and gave way to thankfulness for simply having had Sylvia in our lives. That realization was, for me, the beginning of the healing process. I found that recalling good memories and happy times is often bittersweet, but always full of appreciation for what once was.

Today, when I make routine visits to Sylvia's gravesite, pink rose in hand, her absence still stabs. Even so, I know that she's really not beneath that grassy patch of earth, because when I look up at the wide expanse of sky, I see and feel her there. I visualize her through gossamer clouds on a sunny day, or through swirls of fog, or the beating rain that she so loved to feel on her face. Whenever I cross the Golden Gate Bridge, I see her smiling face in the horizon, and I find myself winking at the sky just to say hello. I bask in the sensation of a response. She exists in the beyond and within my heart, and in the hearts of Maggie, Terri, Gilbert, my children, her cousins, friends and all who loved her as deeply as we did.

On the anniversary of Sylvia's death, or at unexpected moments when something reminds me of her, my throat still thickens and my heart aches. And there are other times that fill my heart with joyful remembrance. For instance, recollections of the early birthday parties, camping, our convalescence after surgery and the times we walked giggling in the rain, are all precious memories that nothing will erase. Sylvia's delight in lifting her face up to the falling rain is as vivid in my mind today as if it'd just happened yesterday. The moments spent sitting on the couch watching television or writing thank-you notes after lunch are cherished times. Visions of Sylvia on water skis, in shorts, in sweat suits, in her cotton-candy-pink *quinceañera* dress, or in saucy hats are ever-present. So many memories in my treasure chest are there to draw on—and I do.

Someone suggested after Sylvia's death that our transplant surgery had, in more tactful words, been a waste. Nothing could be further from the truth. I have not a trace of regret for having gone through the surgery. The opposite is true. The best thing I ever did was to talk Sylvia into permitting me to be her donor, which in the end, allowed me to always be a part of her. It gave her six months of normalcy, a condition only someone who knows what it's like not to be normal can appreciate. It gave us six more months of her, which in itself was worth the surgery. For me, it was such an enriching dimension to my life that I'd repeat the experience in a nanosecond if at all possible.

I've accepted the fact that we lost Sylvia, not as a result of the transplant surgery, but simply from the unpredictability of life. In this case, the sinus infection was the fluke that started her downward spiral. Why that happened is something we'll never know. As Dr. Amend queries in the interview described in the following pages, "Was it the cause or the symptom?" Whatever the case, let me assure you that her gift to me—allowing me to be her kidney donor—was most definitely a gift not wasted.

Thank you, *mija*, for my birthday gift that November.

23

Dr. William Amend's Interview

I started writing about Sylvia and our experience immediately after her death. Chronicling the events became a much-needed cathartic exercise. When finished, I stored the pages away. In the years that followed, I periodically hauled them out to go over them, to expand on some recollection. At first, I could only bear to read a few pages before being overcome with emotion. As time progressed, I drafted the chronology into more of a narrative. Several more drafts later, it melded into the preceding pages. Besides telling you about a wonderful young woman and the euphoric experience of being a live organ donor, it also serves to honor her memory.

Our story doesn't have the typical ending of most transplant stories. Most organ recipients go on to live long and fruitful lives. While that claim can't be made in our case, it remains an accurate description of our experience. And it's mainly Sylvia's, who is, for our family, the "Angel who watches over us."

After the first draft of this work, I became obsessed with going back to UCSF Medical Center to get clear in my mind the causes leading to Sylvia's death. First, I obtained my medical file from UCSF's Records Department. From it, the chronology of events was verified, not to mention the spelling of medical terms.

A desire to speak with Dr. Amend, the nephrologist who had spearheaded Sylvia's care, became a priority. I knew how busy his schedule was, yet I became convinced that, for the purpose of this book, it was vital to get his accounting of what had precipitated Sylvia's final days. It was important not to misconstrue any of the facts. I realized that at the time of her hospitalization, my attempts to be objective and to absorb medical facts were handicapped by emotion. My recollection of events could have been skewed by personal feelings, and I was concerned about this.

Dr. Amend graciously consented to meet with me. It was an exciting development, and I couldn't wait to hear his professional account. One fall, I reported to the UCSF Transplant Surgery and Transplant Nephrology Department to meet with him. The windowed hallway on the floor of his office was immediately familiar from the early days of my testing to become a donor. Though a bit nervous, I forced myself to remain calm enough to carry on a rational, unemotional conversation. Because of his busy schedule, I'd prepared some notes to economize as much of his time as possible and to guide me through the interview.

The minute he came out to the reception area, I recognized him, much like seeing a dear friend after many years. He was of medium height, trim, nearing retirement age, and walked with a brisk gait probably honed by years of navigating through hospital hallways. After he greeted me, we walked down the hall. We entered his small office, and I sat in one of two chairs facing his desk. I thought of the people who must have sat, and will continue to sit, in the same spot to hear good, bad or devastating news. I felt comfortable in the room, sensing hope and compassion within its walls. That was probably due in no small part to Dr. Amend.

He immediately convinced me that he truly remembered Sylvia and her family, which is astonishing in view of the number of people he must have dealt with. He asked about Maggie, Terri and Gilbert. After exchanging small talk, I explained the purpose of my visit.

"Doctor, as I mentioned to you over the telephone, I'm writing a book about Sylvia and my experience with the transplant surgery. It's really important to me to have it end on a hopeful note and emphasize the benefit of being a live donor rather than dwelling on the fact that she died. I'm comforted by the fact that the surgery gave her six months of quality living that she wouldn't have had otherwise. And as you know, she was able to go without dialysis during those months, return to work and carry on in a normal fashion. But to begin with, I feel I need to establish a clear picture in my mind as to exactly what happened to reverse her earlier progress. She seemed to be doing so well after surgery. I'd like to get your view of the medical aspects that led to her death so I can better understand the totality of it all."

I've been accused of sounding too businesslike at times, and this was probably such an instance. Aside from not taking too much of his time, I wanted to get right to the point.

Dr. Amend rested his hands on the desk before starting. "I had her file pulled and looked it over to refresh my memory." He fingered the manila folder before him, but never opened it, as if brief referral to its contents had freshened total recall. Adjusting himself in his chair, he spoke in a deliberate, moderate tone, looking me straight in the eye the whole time while I took notes.

"Sylvia contracted an intractable poly-infection which actually consisted of three infections, or a poly-infectious condition. The primary infection was a virus known as CMV, which affects transplant recipients in particular—all transplant recipients, not only kidney patients. It's the ultimate fear of transplant patients and their doctors. What this virus does is set up lung and kidney conditions that make fighting other conditions worse. As years progress, it's becoming less serious, partly because drug companies have developed prophylactics, medicines resulting in less chance of CMV development, as in Sylvia's case.

"Then, she developed a lung bacterial infection which damaged her respiratory system. On top of that, the third complication was the development of a fungal infection, aspergillus, whose treatment is only successful approximately three percent of the time. That's an exceedingly low stat. The situation resulted in an iniquitous, or an all-pervading, situation which was addressed with an antibacterial cocktail treatment, or a combination of medicines designed to attack all three components of the poly-infection condition."

As an aside, he touched on how the drug and biotech companies have developed more effective drugs since Sylvia's ordeal and how current and future patients might fare better because of these advances. Apparently, with each succeeding year, new discoveries are made that mitigate and overcome such infections.

When he finished with this explanation, I asked, "Was it the sinus infection that started all this in motion?"

Without hesitation, he answered, "It may only have been a symptom, versus a cause, of the start of the CMV infection. It's hard to say."

Holding out his hands, flipping one palm over, then back, he said, "Cause or symptom?" This gesture eloquently demonstrated that either conclusion could be correct. Perhaps both had conspired together. "Who knows?" he added.

It was tremendously important for me to identify the trigger that had started Sylvia's problems. Originally, we'd all thought that the medication originally given to her for a sinus infection was ineffectual due to the immunosuppressants she had had to take as a transplant organ recipient. And because of this ineffectiveness, the sinus infection had raged uncontained, causing the complications that led to her last hospital stay. Now I had learned that the sinus infection might have merely been a symptom, not the cause of her downward spiral—a critical difference to my previous understanding and one that I was pleased to have clarified.

There was another reason his explanations held such importance for me. Deep in my psyche, I'd suppressed an inner fear ever since Sylvia's death. What if my kidney had been defective in some way? Had it been too old? Not good enough? I had to ask. "Is it possible, Dr. Amend, that there was something wrong with my kidney? That somehow it didn't do the proper job?"

The speed of his answer served to quickly dispel that nagging fear. "No, not at all. That would have been detected during or immediately after surgery. No, that wasn't an issue."

With lighter shoulders, I resumed my shorthand. He took a moment to explain the new surgery techniques that have made live organ donation easier. Today, instead of one large incision of approximately six to seven inches, surgeons make four small incisions. He held up his fingers, pinching together about an inch and a half distance. Micro-surgery techniques make it possible to go in to disconnect and cauterize the arteries and veins leading to and from the organ via these small incisions. They then cut a small slit above the pubic bone and extract the kidney through that. This results in less trauma to the donor's body and less recuperation time—approximately three weeks versus the six weeks it took when I had the surgery. I was amazed at the improvements. It was easy to appreciate how much simpler and less invasive the newer techniques were.

He returned to Sylvia's case. "You must understand that the poly-infectious condition impacted her body so much that all her energies were necessarily devoted to fighting off these organisms. Such a struggle can impact the will to live simply due to the sheer exhaustion associated with such a concentrated effort."

That helped explain Sylvia's apparent inertia during her last hospitalization. Her usual fighting spirit was gone. Could her body and spirit have been basically fatigued? From what I was hearing, it sounded plausible.

He leaned back in his chair, shifting to a different approach. Offering his own insight, he reflected on a different aspect of doctoring.

"I find that, sooner or later, the patient almost expresses to their physician, perhaps through eye contact or some other method, that the care of the family be taken over by the doctor. Older doctors, and some younger ones with that insight, see that everything medically possible for the patient is being done by everyone concerned—the fine transplant nurses, staff members, etc. The doctors and staff, of course, are more familiar with the patient's health, not necessarily the family members. There comes a time when, by looking into a patient's eyes, one can discern that what is desired by the patient is support and attention to his or her family. It's a common occurrence to receive such an indication."

As if I wouldn't believe him, he cited our situation. "In Sylvia's case, I turned my attention to Maggie. For example, one day in the waiting room, Maggie, through her tears, briefly touched on a recollection of the playful moments between Armando and Sylvia and how much Sylvia loved her father. At that juncture, I snatched the opportunity to draw this subject matter out of her so she'd recall the happier moments Sylvia had experienced in life. And as additional reminiscences surfaced, she was able to laugh. In the midst of such worry, Maggie was able to actually laugh about the good times screening through her memory, each triggering a subsequent good memory. This was part of the attempt to carry out Sylvia's implied wish that Maggie be comforted."

Dr. Amend watched me as I scribbled onto my pad, wanting to be sure I understood. My notebook captured his exact words because I actually did grasp their full import.

He continued, "I think this capability is a gift that needs to be nourished. I deal with people on all different levels. In instances like Sylvia's, it isn't pleasant telling people the facts."

Dr. Amend further elaborated on how using this ability appeals to people's beliefs in an afterlife, and that it also assists resignation to the possibility of their loved one's death. He believes that this is a God-given gift and one that he tries to foster because of the positive effects— despite the bleak circumstance requiring its application. In his opinion, it's just as important as attending to the physical needs of the patient. He was obviously proud of possessing this skill, not for his own edification, but for the assistance he genuinely feels it renders to the patients' families.

He also noted that sometimes, after interacting in this way with a family (presumably, after delivering bad news), members of that family might pass him in the hallway and see him joking with another person, smiling or laughing. Although he is aware that this might be hurtful to them, the reality is that he must go on and do what he can for others. It's not that he lacks sensitivity. Rather, it affirms a commitment to keep doctoring in the face of all that doctoring entails.

Having experienced his method firsthand, I can attest to its effectiveness. Though I couldn't appreciate it at the time, in looking back, I truly got a sense that all that could be done was indeed done. We never doubted the extraordinary care Sylvia received from the doctors and nurses. It could not have been finer.

When he finished sharing the medical details that I'd requested and detailed his "formula" for interacting with families in situations such as ours, I realized, as I sat in his small office that offered such hope and compassion, that I was satisfied to the depth of my soul.

"Thank you for your time, doctor. I know how busy you are, and I really appreciate this opportunity."

He accompanied me back to the reception desk, gave me his card and asked what the title of the book was going to be. At that time, the title was going to be simply *Sylvia*. However, sometime after this interview, a best-seller by that name honored another memorable lady, Sylvia Plath. So the original title had to be scratched in favor of the present one. As it turns out, I think it's more appropriate.

I thanked him profusely for meeting with me. When I left the enormous UCSF Medical Center complex, it was with a lighter tread and a burden lifted. I felt a tremendous gratitude for its existence.

Concluding this interview was the final component I needed to complete the book. It also closed an important chapter in my life. Without realizing it at the time, it also cracked open a door to a wholly different world.

24

The Case for Organ Donation

For those considering being a live donor of a kidney, liver or lung, I sincerely hope that they concentrate on the success of Sylvia's and my surgery rather than the circumstance of her death. That was a tragedy. Given today's medical progress, it might have been avoided. Advances in surgical procedures and medications, especially in the area of immuno-suppressants, improve organ transplantation every day, as noted in the interview with Dr. William Amend. Kidney recipients can expect the lifespan of a transplanted organ to be twenty years plus, and even that is expanding. Ten years ago, that lifespan was only thirteen years.

I like to dwell on the pre-surgery, surgery, post-surgery and recuperation moments related to our surgery. They were exciting and hopeful times. When I think of Sylvia, I remember her as she looked when healthy. But immersing myself into the task of writing was still not enough to fill the void left by her absence. It unnerved me to think that the surgery had been so successful, only to have her die.

Even as I asked God for comfort and acknowledged His will, my soul ached with pain. Not that it shook my faith. I often recalled a quote the Sisters of Mercy, my high school teachers, had asked us to remember. "Dear God, since you've sent me this cross, please grant me the strength to bear it." They assured us we'd never be given anything more than we could handle. It had sustained me when I went through my divorce, so I knew it to be true. My trust in Him never faltered.

Eventually I concluded that there really is no end to someone's life. His or her influence lingers like an exquisite fragrance deeply embedded in one's senses. While I could no longer see, hear or touch Sylvia, it didn't mean that she wasn't with us. Still, the constant sense of her spirit continued to nag at me. It wasn't enough to be thankful for having had her in our lives. I couldn't leave it at just that. An inner disquiet lingered. I had a looming sense of being on the brink of a new Sylvia experience that I couldn't shake off. Like a premonition.

Finally, a door cracked open and allowed a sliver of light, of insight. It drew me to it. Curious, I opened it and crossed over its threshold. In doing that, I discovered a means to honor Sylvia's memory. It was as if she had led me by the hand toward a new mission. It showed me the way to not only commemorate her life, but to promote gifting life to others. I now share what followed from that experience, keeping in mind that it is she who inspired it.

I discovered the National Kidney Foundation's (NKF) volunteer program called Healthy Kidneys For Life and signed up to go to elementary schools to promote the program. It's aimed at fifth graders and emphasizes the importance of exercise and nutrition to maintain healthy kidneys. In an era when obesity among our young children is skyrocketing, the program is timely and relevant. I found going to classrooms filled with fifth graders both fun and stimulating.

Using a mock-up model of the kidney, the program volunteers explain its function and the critical role it plays in maintaining good health. Development of good eating habits that restrict the intake of salt, fats and sugar is discussed while displaying the latest food pyramid charts. Drinking lots of water, going to the bathroom when you first feel the urge to do so, and avoiding illegal drugs, tobacco and alcohol are also covered. But the main thrust is to encourage a healthy lifestyle that promotes healthy kidneys. Students seem fascinated by the presentation. A question and answer period follows, and their questions usually reflect thoughtful consideration of the subject. I think it's a great program and was pleased to be associated with it.

After being introduced to the NKF, I learned of another organization—the California Transplant Donor Network (CTDN)—and also began volunteering for them. It's an Organ Procurement Organization (OPO) and their mission statement is: "The California Transplant Donor Network saves and improves lives through organ and tissue donation for transplantation." That in a nutshell is a simplified description of their important role in saving lives through their Donate Life objective. Volunteers help carry out that mission by assisting in community education, predisposing people to the idea, spreading the word, and encouraging people to sign up on the registry via their website (please see Resources Page in the Epilogue).

CTDN belongs to the United Network for Organ Sharing (UNOS), as does every other OPO in the country. In 1984 Congress passed the National Organ Transplant Act to address the critical shortage of deceased donor organs in this country. UNOS was established to form a national organ matching system as a non-profit scientific and educational organization. It administers the nation's Organ Procurement and Transplantation Network. This includes collecting and managing data about every transplant event in the U.S., maintaining the organ waiting lists, facilitating the organ matching and placement process, and development of a national organ transplantation policy with input from medical professionals, transplant recipients and donor families. Community education about their operation is one of their priorities. CTDN and every other OPO are required to follow UNOS regulations. Every hospital has an OPO assigned to it. The OPO coordinates efforts to ensure a smooth donation process. All this was news to me. When I did find out about them and their commitment, I didn't hesitate to join their volunteer group.

Working with the NKF and CTDN in honor of Sylvia's memory is now an important element in my life. At first, volunteering was a means to ease my grief. But the more I learned about the work they do, the more it drew me in. Helping to spread the word on how to save lives, either by encouraging healthy habits or promoting organ donation, was the purpose I needed to commemorate Sylvia's life. My small contribution of time has brought me incredible insight into the potential we all have to save lives. So, in this post era of Sylvia's life, I owe her another thank you for again gifting me with an opportunity to receive more than I have given.

It's an amazing capability to be able to extend someone's life by donating an organ. Fortunately, a kidney can come from a live donor who, other than the temporary interval of recovery, suffers no impediment to his or her health. And surgical methods are improving daily, shortening the recuperation time. The same holds true for liver and lung donations from live donors who are able to function normally post-surgery.

The subject of live organ donation usually surfaces only when an immediate family member is diagnosed as being in need of a transplant. It seems that it's not until our own lives are touched with a loved one's organ failure that we become aware of the transplant possibility. I know I never considered it until Sylvia's second rejection. Without a doubt, it's a blessed alternative to subjecting someone to the indeterminable period of time associated with being on the organ waiting lists. In essence, a family can be a private donor pool *if* they choose to look at themselves that way.

However, because of the enormous potential for abuse with living organ donation, organ transplant organizations are very cautious about promoting it, although they definitely support it. CTDN was quick to acknowledge my experience as a living donor. Interestingly, the reaction from fellow volunteers is more effusive. This is probably because many of them have been recipients. While CTDN's orientation sessions confirm their support and appreciation for living donation, their efforts concentrate on organ donation after death.

Naturally, it's important that the decision to be a living donor is free from coercion or guilt. Doctors and transplant units are extremely sensitive to a patient's ability to secure a live donation and advise him or her and their family of that option. Other than that, no pressure is placed on the patient to solicit family members, or on family members to offer. Additionally, the psychiatric portion of the donor's qualification process is geared to insure that the donation is made freely, without promise of compensation or gain and simply out of altruistic motives.

It's astounding to note that today there are 98,000 people on organ transplant waiting lists in the United States. Over 70 percent are kidney patients. The average waiting time is up to six years. That's an incredibly long time to wait when one's life is in jeopardy. Every day 18-20 people die because their turns did not materialize. From the approximately 2.5 million deaths yearly in the U.S., only fourteen thousand of those registered as organ donors qualify to be donors. That is a miniscule percentage, which is why OPOs are anxious to cast the net wide to achieve greater registration numbers. Names on these lists are expected to double within the next ten years, according to current projections made by the NKF. This is another reason encouragement to register for organ donation after death has become such a high priority.

Registration as an organ donor is being supported not only by national organ donor organizations and the NKF, but also by agencies like the Department of Motor Vehicles, who facilitate driver registration on the donor registry. Not only can you have your wish to be an organ donor clearly indicated on your driver's license, but you are now able to go online to a special national registry that will document your desire to be an organ donor. Check your local DMV office for their online registry.

We don't have a cure for cancer, Parkinson's, multiple sclerosis or cystic fibrosis, to name but a few diseases. Yet it is definitely within our power to save the lives of those 98,000 on the waiting list. We have the solution; all we need to do is apply it. We are walking, breathing lifesavers and possess the capability to gift life to those suffering from chronic organ failure. If more of us would register, it has been estimated that we could eliminate the waiting lists within ten years. To all who are aware of and appalled by the throngs waiting their turns on lengthy organ recipient lists, such a result would be music to their ears. Hear and take to heart that we can make this prediction a reality.

Many people don't normally think about becoming organ donors. Others feel uncomfortable with the subject. It's simply not an everyday topic. In that respect, I was certainly normal. It never occurred to me to be a live donor until my own daughter volunteered herself for Sylvia's benefit. I credit Cynthia with my own mental awakening to the realization that I could gift life. I'd like to emphasize that my decision to advocate this cause doesn't mean that I dwell on death. Rather, it's the realization that eight lives can be saved through the donated organs of just one person. Since my last day on earth is eventually inevitable, it makes sense to me to donate life to others.

I can assure you that if someone you love became affected by organ failure, you'd be astounded at how much information is available on the subject. Both the NKF and OPO organizations offer an abundance of free educational material that is readily available for the asking. Remember that no question is insignificant. You'd be pleasantly surprised at how many informative and willing personnel in this field are ready to give you whatever you need to make educated decisions regarding organ donation.

For example, one of the many questions I had during the early stages of qualifying as a living donor was about age. Is age a factor for being a donor? At the time, I was fifty-four, hiking with the Sierra Club, healthy and very energetic. Yet I wondered if I was past the suitable age for qualifying. The transplant clinic and everything I read on the matter conveyed a resounding "No!" Availing yourself of the information and material disbursed by transplant clinics, NKF and OPOs will satisfy your every question.

Recently, I've noticed greater media coverage of this topic. We often read about donor and recipient cases in the newspapers or hear about them on the news. But these stories are quickly forgotten. It's understandable. So much goes on in our lives today that in self-defense, we only permit a certain amount of information to filter in. Here are some of the more memorable stories I've heard or read about.

A radio report I heard in May of 2004 related to my question on age. A seventy-six-year-old woman in the state of Oregon became the successful living donor for her adult daughter. Another example: R. C. Owens, the famous former San Francisco Forty-Niner football player, received a kidney transplant at the age of 69 in 2004. In 2005, comedian George Lopez received a kidney donation from his wife. Aren't we an amazing species to be able to gift life to one another in this manner?

The grandmother and the football player mentioned above attest to the fact that being young is not a requirement for being either a donor or a recipient. Naturally, being healthy is. But I believe that more of us are becoming more conscious of what healthful habits are and attempting to incorporate them into our lives.

It should be noted that both the African American and the Latino communities have high occurrence rates for kidney failure due to high diabetes rates in their ethnic groups. Diabetes is the leading cause of kidney failure. A terrible statistic reported in the *San Francisco Chronicle* claims that in 2003, while as many as 4,334 African Americans received an organ transplant, 1,495 died waiting. The Latino community is similarly affected by these adverse statistics. Ethnic groups are especially targeted by the NKF and OPOs due to these high organ failure rates. CTDN cites on their website, "Education is also targeted towards improving awareness of organ and tissue donation in our various communities including African-American, Latino, Chinese, Filipino and Vietnamese populations…. Our staff has developed language-specific and culturally-appropriate materials regarding organ and tissue donation and the success of transplantation." Both NKF and OPOs print materials in a variety of languages as part of their commitment to ethnic communities.

In my opinion, reducing the number of names on the lengthy organ waiting lists should be one of the nation's highest priorities. The *Reno Gazette* featured an article in the January 5, 2005 Investment Section of their newspaper which stated, "The critical shortage of organs for people awaiting transplants long has vexed policymakers and doctors." The article mentions that tax breaks for organ donation are being considered in some states, as well as legislation to encourage live and deceased organ donations. The article continues to state that "the Organ Donation and Recovery Improvement Act authorizes federal grants to states, transplant centers and other entities to help cover living donors' non-medical expenses."

Undoubtedly, these are steps in the right direction. But when one recalls the thousands of names on organ waiting lists, it is clear that more needs to be done. We cannot ignore the many who die waiting their turn when we have a viable solution within our grasp. There's no question that we need to do more and can do more. We have the resources to do so. It is within our power to save lives—let's do it!

When I learned that "one deceased person can save eight lives," CTDN had my attention. Then they added, "If you add tissue and bone marrow donation, that number increases to over fifty lives." What an astounding fact! Think of it. Eight persons or even more can live if one person chooses to be an organ donor. Organ waiting lists can become a thing of the past if we all take to heart and embrace the CTDN slogan, "Donate Life."

The mechanics of donating organs at the time of death are expertly and compassionately handled by the OPOs assigned to each hospital. By law, hospitals must report cases of imminent brain death. Such notification automatically places a clinical coordinator from the hospital's OPO at the scene to offer grief counseling and aid families in coordinating the issue of organ donation. They also assist in a variety of other ways; e.g. notifying other family members or friends of the death, privacy protection from the media if requested, assistance with mortuary arrangements—even with transport of a body to another geographical region—and coordinating efforts with embassies to ship the deceased to a country of origin.

Grief counseling, general comfort and support with issues that arise during the difficult time of losing a loved one are of paramount importance to every OPO. Everything possible that can be done for the donor family is provided. I know this to be true from personal feedback from donor families and from hearing scores of examples during our volunteer orientation sessions. One of the strongest assertions OPOs make is that their number one priority is the donor family.

The clinical coordinator contributes a high level of sensitivity to a family's needs. Aside from supporting families during their crises, they are in charge of obtaining the necessary consent forms and documentation from the family so that the process of organ donation can go forward smoothly. They are genuinely concerned with the grief the patient's family are going through and provide as much solace as they can.

In the summer of 2005, I attended a CTDN volunteer training session, and several speakers addressed the group. One was Mark, a clinical coordinator who had most recently coordinated the organ donation from a thirteen-year-old Boy Scout who'd been killed while on a backpacking trip at Sequoia National Park in California. This coordinator had just returned from the Fresno area and was visibly drained from the emotionally-charged event. The parents of the Boy Scout had discussed organ donation in front of both their sons just weeks before the tragedy. As a result, there was no equivocation about the donation of organs after the fatal accident occurred. In the next day's newspaper article the father is quoted, "When it came up … at the hospital yesterday, there was never any question about donating the organs."

Mark detailed the support he was able to render to the family, how he shielded them from the media at their request, and the expression of gratitude they extended him at his departure. During a final embrace from the young boy's mother, she thanked him for all his efforts and told him that she didn't think she could have gone through it all without him. He freely admitted to crying with the family and couldn't praise them enough for their courage and foresight. It was one of the most poignant moments at the orientation session. At the epicenter of what no family should have to go through, human generosity triumphed and others were saved. My mind couldn't help imagining the utter joy on that day of all the recipients that this family had given life to.

It's a fact that many families who honor the expressed wishes of their loved ones to be organ donors are filled with an inner tranquility. OPOs state that such families frequently experience a tremendous sense of comfort in knowing that they have complied with their loved one's last wishes. Many even express a profound lessening of their sorrow knowing that a part of their beloved continues to exist through the recipients.

Every year, CTDN hosts an event to honor those families of organ donors from the previous year who wish to be acknowledged. The recipients and their families are also invited. Every year, numerous recipients take the opportunity to say "thank you" to donor families and those in the audience who assisted in the effort. The *San Francisco Chronicle* wrote about one particular event in their April 25, 2004 edition. It cited one of the recipients, a four-year-old girl who shyly addressed the crowd of 1,400 to say "Thank you for saving my life" to the donor family. Because of their benevolence, she would be attending kindergarten in the fall. The article also stated that there were few dry eyes when she spoke.

In another instance, the father of a young adolescent who lost his life when struck by a hit-and-run driver while riding his bicycle is quoted as saying, "It's not a hard decision to make. It's just a hard time to make any decisions." Once that father and his family met one of the recipients of their son's organs at this event and witnessed the results of their decision, they were able to reconcile, in part, their tragedy. It enabled them to draw something positive from their loss. They were, as were all the donor families present, awarded the "Star of Life," a silver necklace with a red rose as a symbol of gratitude from CTDN. The Star of Life was designed by a woman who received life from a donor family.

The mother of a young boy who'd died as a result of a freak skate-boarding accident admitted that signing the donation papers had been difficult. Her immediate reaction to the OPO coordinator who approached her at the hospital was, "Vultures!" But when she heard that a five-month-old baby had been saved from imminent death, she changed her mind and was gratified to know that a part of her son lived on.

Typically, when people who agonized about the decision to donate the organs of their loved one can see and speak with the persons their decision affected, they are grateful for being instrumental in saving their lives. Such meetings are of invaluable comfort. This brings to mind a very important aspect of becoming an organ donor. Discuss the decision with your family and loved ones. This cannot be overemphasized. It is, in fact, one of the most critical and essential elements to insure that your expressed wish to gift life is carried out. At the time of death, families may be afraid of doing the wrong thing or are too bereft to think clearly. They may misunderstand the process. Perhaps they think it desecrates the body in some way or leaves it disfigured. It does not. They may be under the mistaken impression that there is a cost associated with the surgery required for organ removal—not so.

They may believe that their religion prohibits such donation. None of the major religions object to live or deceased organ donation. You'll find that the brochures of all the agencies listed here have direct quotes from most religions supporting organ donation, from previous Pope John XXIII, to rabbis, ministers, clergy and other religious representatives. (Please refer to Religious Reference in Epilogue.) It's encouraging to note that the current pope, Pope Benedict XVI, is the first organ donor card-carrying pope.

The only known group that CTDN and I found in our research that doesn't support organ donation is gypsies. They believe that their bodies and spirits remain connected in some way for a full year after death. As a result, they do not wish to disturb that link. It's a belief that must be respected. But other than that group, our research could not come up with any other religion that did not support organ donation.

Families who are concerned about having open caskets during funeral services often ask about signs of visible evidence that organs have been removed. There is none. More importantly, the same respect and care shown to a live donor is extended to a deceased person. The word "cadaver" is no longer used because a person does not cease to be a person after death and, therefore, is referred to as a deceased *person*. The medical field, all OPOs and NKF affirm that a deceased person continues to deserve the same level of respect as when he or she was alive.

The deceased donor is not carelessly treated. For example, surgical openings are stitched closed. If the deceased is a bone donor and the bone removed happens to be the longest bone in the arm, a prosthesis will be attached so that an open casket viewing remains possible and the arm will appear to be normal. If skin tissue is donated, none is taken from areas that would be visible in an open casket. Everyone involved in the coordination of this process is highly cognizant of the enormous gift that organ donation represents, and their appreciation knows no bounds.

All these questions and more can be thoroughly answered by the OPO's clinical coordinator assigned to your particular hospital. They are mentioned here to illustrate the degree of care and respect that every deceased person receives during the process of organ donation.

25

A Prime Example of Selfless Love

There are many thousands of heart-rending stories involving organ donation. One donor family's experience impressed me deeply, and I want to share it with you.

In early 2008, the Zaragoza family, who'd been referred to me by the CTDN, agreed to tell me the story of how their son, Matthew, died and about their decision to donate his organs. It was as if Providence had led me to this extraordinary home at this particular time. Hearing their story not only validated, but fortified my opinion of the power we all have to save lives.

I arrived at a nice residential neighborhood in Manteca, California, on a Saturday afternoon. The sign above the doorbell amused me: "Forget the dog, beware of the kids!" I needed the smile those words prompted, because I was a bit nervous about the interview. I was concerned about not saying anything to hurt or offend the family.

I had barely had time to shift from one foot to the other when the door swung open. Zona, pronounced Zoona, Zaragoza, a young, blond wife and mother, held the door wide and welcomed me. A pair of piercing blue eyes smiled into mine. "Hi, you must be Bel."

"Yes. Zona? Thanks so much for agreeing to meet with me. I really appreciate it."

"Well, Cathy Olmo told me about you, and I thought it was a great idea." Cathy is the dynamic community coordinator for our local CTDN.

Zona led me into their family room. Cody, a beagle-lab mix, inspected me and responded to my petting, eagerly allowing me to befriend him. Zona introduced me to her eighteen-year-old daughter, who was sitting at the kitchen counter with her boyfriend, who was eating.

"This is Katrina, Matthew's twin sister. Her boyfriend is on his lunch hour."

Katrina, a petite teenager with medium brown hair and bluish-gray eyes, threw me a warm smile and introduced her boyfriend. He said "Hi" in between bites.

Zona turned into the family room and sat on one corner of the couch. I made myself comfortable on the opposite end, and Cody was quick to snuggle up against me. Two of the other children were not present, twenty-year-old Mark and thirteen-year-old Kristy, eighteen and ten respectively at the time of their brother's death.

I repeated that I was in the process of being published, had heard their story from CTDN, and wanted to include it in one of the book's final chapters, if they agreed. First, I wanted to be sure that I had my facts straight. We exchanged small talk about how great CTDN's support was to families in their situation. I covered a bit of my own background and what had prompted me to write the book. Zona thanked me for including Matthew's story in this book. That comment became the tip of an emotional iceberg whose depth I was just beginning to explore.

Just as Zona started her son's story, her husband, Jose, entered the family room from the sliding glass patio door off their garden. A handsome, dark-haired man with a light complexion and a medium build headed towards me, his hand held out in welcome. After we were introduced, he sat on the raised hearth of the fireplace, facing us. His English is very articulate, although a slight Spanish accent tinges his speech. With my background, it's a pleasant and familiar sound.

"What part of Mexico are you from?" I asked in Spanish.

He said, "Michoacan."

"My family was from Parral, Chihuahua, the north," I said before reverting to English again.

Jose nodded agreeably, and Zona explained to him that she was about to tell me about Matthew. He nodded and lowered his eyes, ready to hear again what he knew by heart. Zona began. My notebook in hand, I prepared to take it all down.

On September 16, 2005, sixteen-year-old Matthew was in the second football varsity game of his life. My immediate thought was that he must have been a pretty good athlete to be playing high-school varsity at his age.

"It was the kick-off return, going in for the tackle, when somehow, an opposing team player and he had a helmet-to-helmet collision." Her cobalt blue eyes got serious as her hands orchestrated the scene. At this point, we were all on the football field. "The other boy continued playing, not realizing that anything had happened and that Matthew was down." Her kind tone revealed that she truly believed it was an unintentional, freak accident. "Matthew didn't get back up," she went on. "The coaches rushed out to the field."

Jose interjected, "I ran onto the field and saw him lying on the ground. The coaches and medical staff told me to hold back, but I knelt beside him and held his hand. I said, 'Don't worry, *mijo*, everything is going to be all right.' I sensed it was bad as he looked up at me. While I held his hand, he closed his eyes."

Zona tried to reach Matthew, but was held back at the sidelines with Kristy, the younger daughter. "I knew right away that Matthew had gone down, and I could tell by the way the emergency crew were working on him that something was very wrong."

Twin sister Katrina was a cheerleader and had been cheering her school team and brother on. When the collision occurred, someone said they thought it was Matthew. Katrina knew someone had gone down, but at first she didn't think it was her brother. The paramedics had arrived and weren't letting anyone get close to Matthew. The only reason Jose was permitted to remain beside his son was because he was already there. Zona, Kristy, Katrina and friends watched anxiously from the sidelines. Someone suggested they hold hands in prayer.

"I can still vividly remember joining hands in prayer." Zona paused as if screening the scene across her memory.

"Where did they take him?" I asked.

"San Joaquin General Hospital. Jose was permitted to accompany Matthew in the ambulance, but me and the kids were driven separately to the hospital by friends. We waited while they tried to stabilize him in the emergency room. The neurosurgeon told us that he was surprised at the extent of cerebral damage." Zona went on to describe the seriousness of Matthew's head injuries. They were not typical of a football injury of this type. On a scale from one to ten, ten being the most serious, Matthew's injuries were diagnosed as a nine.

She said, "Usually, they don't operate for his kind of injuries, but the doctor said that because Matthew was so young and healthy, he felt he could take the risk. He asked for our consent to perform surgery. We agreed." She leaned back into the cushions and paused before saying, "He never regained consciousness." She needed to dab her eyes with a tissue before continuing. Jose eyes were moist. He sat on the hearth, outwardly still, but obviously roiling within.

After a week on life support, Matthew was declared brain dead by two physicians. The Zaragozas sought one more opinion from another doctor just because they felt they needed to. When the third opinion was the same, they knew they had to withdraw life support.

I glanced at Jose, who was looking at his wife. Their eyes reflected the heavy weight of that decision. "He died on September 23rd," Zona said quietly. "After one week on life support. He was sixteen years, six months and twenty-three days old."

Between tears and smiles, I heard about Matthew the athlete, the jokester, the happy son, the hefty eater. They brought up remembrances, offering tiny details that are deeply etched in their memories.

Switching back to the hospital scene, Zona talked about the coordinator who first approached them about donating Matthew's organs. "He never mentioned that he, himself, was an organ recipient. We didn't learn about that until much later." The coordinator had received either a kidney or a liver, they weren't sure which. But both Zona and Jose were impressed with the coordinator's sensitivity at not mentioning that fact. "Otherwise, we might have felt some pressure," Zona said. They also felt the coordinator had the utmost respect and compassion for their situation throughout each phase of their ordeal.

After their discussion with the coordinator, Zona asked Jose if he wanted to donate Matthew's organs. He responded, "Definitely."

At this point, Jose edged forward from the hearth to say in his soft voice, "I only wished that I had heard Matthew say that he wanted to donate his organs. I would have liked to have heard it from HIM, that's all." A tormented expression appeared on his kindly face. "Otherwise, I thought it was the right thing to do."

Once they had agreed to donate Matthew's organs, they went to their bishop for counsel before discussing it with their children.

"What faith is that?" I asked

Zona replied, "LDS, the Church of Latter Day Saints."

I shared my research regarding religious attitudes towards organ donations and told them that the majority of religions support organ donation. She nodded, saying they'd been given ample support and comfort from their bishop. His guidance gave them confidence to seek their children's views. The decision to donate Matthew's organs became a unanimous family decision. Zona and Jose were thankful for that bittersweet unity of purpose they shared. It was obvious that their children's support meant a great deal to them. Mark, Katrina and Kristy agreed that donating their brother's organs was the right thing to do. A few weeks later, I would see and hear them say as much on *The Montel Williams Show*.

I asked, "Backing up a bit, at what point were you approached by the OPO?"

Jose told me that Zona's brother was an RN at San Joaquin General and that he had prepared them beforehand about the possibility of being contacted by the OPO if Matthew were declared brain dead. "He realized more fully just how serious Matthew's situation was," Zona added.

"At first, he was against our consenting to donate Matthew's organs," Jose said. Later, Zona's brother did agree with their decision. Zona suggested that his initial opposition was probably due to the shock that his nephew was dying. When he had given it further thought, he came around to their way of thinking.

Zona explained more about the first contact by the CTDN clinical coordinator. "It's only after two doctors declare someone brain dead that you can be asked about donating the organs. Like I said, we went ahead on our own and got a third opinion simply because we wanted to." Then she added with a quiet finality, "All that could possibly be done was done. We know that."

Both Jose and Zona emphasized that they were confident that everything possible is done to save the life of someone who is on life support. I'd heard that many times, but it was very satisfying to hear it confirmed by someone's actual experience. Zona said, and Jose agreed, that during the entire time of Matthew's struggle, they had received incredible support from everyone—the schools, the trauma team, the doctors and hospital staff. Family and friends rallied around them. Their praise for the CTDN coordinator and the hospital staff was especially generous.

They touched on a couple of coincidences that surrounded Matthew's accident. Both seemed to have made a deep impression on them. For them, these additional twists of fate added to the extraordinary circumstance of their tragedy. Ironically, the opposing team member who had collided with Matthew was celebrating his birthday on that Friday afternoon of the game. The second coincidence described by Zona was, "Matthew was declared brain dead at the exact time of the following week's Friday night high school football kickoff. I always imagine he drifted into the heavens as the national anthem was being sung."

The lump in my throat thickened. I noticed, as she wiped away her tears, that the retelling of Matthew's death was bittersweet. The warm recollection of their beloved son was in a way comforting despite the pain of their loss. Making the decision to donate their son's organs had eased their loss. The entire Zaragoza family were convinced that their Matthew would have approved of their decision to donate his organs, especially when shortly after making that decision, they were aware of the gifts of life they had bequeathed to four other persons.

"There's something I really want to emphasize," Zona said. "Something I want everybody to know. The hospital and coordinator kept us posted when a recipient was identified, when they were going in for the transplant, and if it had been successful. We were really excited for them. It's an indescribable feeling."

Both recalled how sharing in the process had helped in their struggle with Matthew's death. With each completed transplantation surgery, their joy of gifting life through Matthew grew to renewed heights. They claimed that words are simply inadequate to express the exhilaration they felt knowing that, because of Matthew, these individuals were brought back from the brink of death. Each notification lifted their spirits. Exchanging warm smiles, the Zaragozas repeated their conviction that Matthew still lives through the four recipients.

At first, they were unaware of the recipients' names. It is the policy of all OPOs not to reveal the names of the recipients unless they receive permission to do so. This also holds true for the donor's family, who may not wish to be identified. Months later, when Jose and Zona did learn their names and actually met the recipients, the entire experience took on even greater meaning.

Four people received seven of Matthew's organs. A fifty-seven-year-old male received one kidney; a forty-seven-year-old male received one kidney and a pancreas; a thirty-nine-year-old African-American woman received his heart and both lungs; and a seventeen-year-old girl received his liver. These four are alive today because of the love the Zaragoza family have (yes, present tense) for their son Matthew and for humanity. In different ways and with different expressions, Zona and Jose affirm that Matthew lives on within the people he gifted life to. Who can argue with that?

Jose asked, "Would you like to see his picture?"

"Absolutely," I said.

By this time, Katrina's boyfriend had left to return to work, and she was quietly sitting behind us in another corner of the room, listening to every word of our conversation.

Jose got up to retrieve a large poster. As he proudly raised it for me to view, a handsome teenager dressed in full football regalia looked out confidently from the frame. He had Jose's dark hair and Zona's light complexion. It's hard to identify whose smile he had inherited, as they both have beautiful smiles. The casual stance of the young athlete, football in one hand, reminded me of a young Joe Montana.

I looked at Katrina, his twin, and compared her petite stature with Matthew's sturdy, athletic build. What contrasting sizes. Yet when I looked at their features, the similarities were there. The identical beaming eyes, the dazzling smiles, and the vibrant demeanor confirmed them as fraternal twins.

Tucked into the four corners of the frame were smaller pictures of the four organ recipients. Their happy expressions reflect the appreciation and benefits of the gift of life they received from Matthew. Zona pointed to each photo and gave a brief rundown on them.

When she finished, I turned to Katrina and said, "This must have really been hard on you, Katrina. I have twin sisters and know how tight twins can be. How did you feel after the accident?"

She was quick to answer. "Yeah, it was awful. When my parents said they wanted to talk to us and that they wanted to talk to me first, I felt a lot of pressure. When they told me what they were thinking of doing, it was really hard. But I couldn't say no because I think Matthew would have agreed with it."

"Do you think about him a lot, feel his presence?" I asked.

"I don't feel his presence so much, but I do dream about him. I dream about him a lot." After an introspective moment, she added, "It was really hard when Mom started getting his clothes together and stuff." I thought she might say something else, but she turned inward and fell silent. The silence and the downcast eyes said it all.

I turned to Zona, who was speaking about CTDN. "Jose volunteers for them now," she said.

Pride showed in his smile as he said that he enjoyed volunteering. Jose and I compared the type of events we volunteered for. We discussed some of the statistics regarding the waiting lists. He corrected my figure of 93,000 patients listed on the waiting lists. "It's now up to 98,000," Jose said. My heart sank at the news and the need to revise my stats.

Toward the end of our interview, the Zaragozas said that Montel, of *The Montel Williams Show* on daytime television, had interviewed them the previous fall and they were waiting to hear when their program would be aired. A week after our interview, she e-mailed me to confirm that their show would be aired on February 12, 2008. I replied that I would be riveted to my TV set and looked forward to seeing it.

By the way, in exchanging e-mails with Zona to set up our meeting, she signed off, "Zona, Jose, Mark, Katrina, Kristy and Matthew in spirit." Matthew will always be with them, with those whose lives he saved, with CTDN, and with all who hear his story.

Our interview lasted about forty-five minutes. Before I left, the three of us hugged several times. Huddling in that family room discussing a horrific tragedy that was turned into a life-saving event for four individuals was a deeply emotional experience. Yes, there's the sorrow of loss. But over that sadness is a balm of solace that their son lives on. And on top of that layer, yet another element enriches their experience. Through their example, they've sown hope for those on the waiting lists and highlighted a cause that merits everyone's attention. What a remarkable family, and what a privilege to have been given the opportunity to meet them.

When I first entered their home, I was already an advocate for organ donation, both living and deceased. On leaving, that commitment was increased tenfold. The Zaragozas epitomize the very message this book hopes to convey. Their story not only validates the cause of organ donation, but is an example of how to live it. Having heard it firsthand was an experience I'll always cherish.

The February 12, 2008 *Montel Williams Show* featured the Zaragozas. I watched it with my sister, Esther, at her house because I wanted someone to share the experience with. Katrina, Jose and Zona sat on the stage with Montel, and Mark and Kristy were in the audience. Mark is now twenty and Kristy thirteen. Katrina, sixteen at the time of the accident, is now eighteen, as is Matthew in their hearts. As Jose and Zona repeated the story I had heard in their family room, there wasn't a dry eye in the audience. Pictures flashed on the screen of the family praying at Matthew's grave, of baby Matthew, and of Matthew and Katrina horsing around. Blurred scenes from a football field with players scrimmaging flashed briefly to accompany Zona's narration, which was punctuated with Jose's comments.

Zona recounted the desperation of those first hours and days after Matthew's accident. She told Montel, "I prayed to God to leave me at least a part of Matthew, even if it meant that I'd have to care for him..." Only a parent could make such an earnest plea.

Montel's expert hosting drew from them the quiet grace of their act, which touched everyone. He asked Katrina about the difficulty of losing a twin and how she had felt on that Friday afternoon.

"It's been crazy. I was actually cheerleading on the field for him. At first I didn't know it was him that went down. Other people in the stands said they thought it was Matthew, but I said I didn't think so." When she realized that it was her brother, she rushed to her mother and Kristy, who were on the sidelines, and watched the medical team work on him.

The cameras panned to Mark and Kristy in the audience as Montel asked them about what they'd thought when their parents asked them about donating Matthew's organs. Mark, another handsome son, said that he encouraged the decision because he knew that it gave Matthew a chance to save other people's lives. Though his lip quivered and eyes glistened, he said it with pride and reaffirmed that through that act, Matthew lived on. Then, recollecting happier times, he added, "Matthew and I shared a bedroom for years. We worked out together every day. He was getting bigger than me and I was getting jealous. I didn't want him to get bigger than me." He laughed at himself, then went on to say that he felt proud that his brother had saved lives, and he knew in his heart that Matthew shared that pride.

Kristy echoed Mark's sentiments. "It makes me happy and has helped me get through the loss and everything. I love that he lives on through other people." To say that Matthew's siblings' words were inspiring is an understatement.

Montel turned to the Zaragozas beside him and asked if they had ever met the recipients of Matthew's organs. They said that they had not. The next moment, that changed.

Tom, now fifty-nine, rushed from the sidelines with arms stretched wide to hug Zona and Jose. Tears flowed. Lorna, now forty-one, followed suit, adding to the tumult. The Zaragozas were hugging part of Matthew, and their jubilation was overpowering. As cameras scanned the audience, a responsive scene of people wiping their tears mirrored the emotions of everyone on the stage. When the camera focused on Mark and Kristy, it showed that they, too, were engulfed in the moment. My sister Esther and I were practically in tears ourselves.

Tom described the frustration of his three-year period on the waiting list, hoping his turn for a kidney transplant would finally materialize. During that time he was on dialysis several times a week. Despite its lifesaving qualities, dialysis had sapped his strength, leaving him listless. He had no energy to participate in life. After receiving Matthew's kidney, he now enjoys life again. He loves to fish and takes his grandchildren fishing. He gratefully acknowledges that his revitalization is due solely to their decision to donate Matthew's organs.

Sitting next to him, Zona clasped Tom's hand firmly with one hand and wiped away persistent tears of joy with the other. With a cracking voice Tom said, "I can't imagine what it would be like to lose one of my kids, and I could tell that Matthew was dearly loved... Because of Matthew, that's why I'm here, and through me, Matthew is still here." He thanked them repeatedly for their loving generosity.

After Lorna's long embrace with Zona and Jose, she said, "I don't have the words to say thank you enough. To live normally and to know that I'll see tomorrow is amazing, and I want to thank you so much. It's awesome to carry on his legacy, and I want you to know that I'm living for *both* of us." Lorna had suffered from congenital heart disease from birth. Her entire life had been plagued with frequent illness, disability and fear of dying. Twice she'd been proclaimed dead after serious heart attacks. Now she enjoys riding a bike and skating, things she never did prior to 2005 when she received Matthew's heart and lungs. The joy of being able to do those two simple activities lit up her eyes as if they were miracles. To her, they were.

As the program's time was running out, a deeply-affected Montel stated, "I have to tell you something. As I sit here and look out on this stage, I see a rainbow. A rainbow of different races and genders." He expressed awe and marveled at how this selfless act had transcended all barriers of age, gender and race. As he shook his head, he reiterated that the Zaragoza family had crossed every barrier to keep people alive. It was almost as if he was astounded that such human generosity was possible. Yet there they sat—living proof that such charitable heights can be achieved. He acknowledged that their example had forced him to consider his opinion of organ donation in a totally different light. In closing he looked over to the Zaragozas and to the recipients and said, "God bless you all."

In April 2008, both Jose and I were part of a volunteer group that helped during CTDN's "In Celebration and Remembrance" ceremony at Chabot College in Hayward. Over 1,700 donor families and recipients attended. We ran into each other by chance and spoke only briefly, as we both had duties in different areas of the event. Jose told me that lots had happened to his family since our January interview. A crew from *The Montel Williams Show* had made a video at their Manteca home for future airing. They'll be representatives of CTDN at the 2009 Rose Bowl Parade float on New Year's Day. And Jose also mentioned that a different media source had expressed an interest in their story. He beamed with pride. I wished we could have talked more, but our workstations needed us. We hugged goodbye and said, "*Adios*." I know it will not be the last time I see him or his family.

On May 12, 2008, *The Montel Williams Show* televised a special show entitled "Finale." It was devoted to the most touching stories of the last season, although Montel hastened to add that it was not in any way a final show and that the summer would see new shows (not repeat episodes). Not surprisingly, the Zaragozas' saga was featured. Scenes of Jose, Zona, Mark, Katrina and Kristy standing in front of Matthew's flower-covered grave and pictures of Matthew in various stages of his life flashed on the screen. Zona spoke for the family. "Seeing the people who received a part of Matthew on your show and being on it was great. We realized that it changed our lives for the best." She said that Montel's show had helped them move further along in the healing process.

The family's appearances on the show are a fitting testimony to what gifting life through organ donation represents. This generous opening of their lives to that cause is a prime example of what selfless love is.

Epilogue

RESOURCES:

The National Kidney Foundation, Inc.
30 East 33rd Street, 11th Floor
New York, NY 10016
(800) 622-9010
www.kidney.org

The National Kidney Foundation of Northern California and Northern
Nevada
131 Steuart Street, Suite 520
San Francisco, CA 94105
(415) 543-3303
www.kidneynca.org

United Network for Organ Sharing (UNOS)
www.unos.org

California Transplant Donor Network
100 Broadway, Suite 600
Oakland, CA 94607
(888) 570-9400
En Español: (800) 588-0024
www.ctdn.org
ww.donateLIFEcalifornia.org

RELIGIOUS VIEWS ON ORGAN DONATIONS:

Golden State Donor Services
"It's About Giving Life"
www.gsds.org

The following is a sampling of official views held by various religions.

AME ZION (AFRICAN METHODIST EPISCOPAL)

Organ and tissue donation is viewed as an act of neighborly love by these denominations. They encourage all members to support donation as a way of helping others.

AMISH

The Amish will consent to transplantation if they believe it is for the well-being of the transplant recipient. John Hostetler, world-renowned authority on Amish religion and professor of anthropology at Temple University in Philadelphia, says in his book, *The Amish Society*, "The Amish believe that since God created the human body, it is God who heals." However, nothing in the Amish understanding of the Bible forbids them from using modern medical services, including surgery, hospitalization, dental work, anesthesia, blood transfusions, or immunization.

ASSEMBLY OF GOD

The church has no official policy regarding organ and tissue donation. The decision to donate is left up to the individual. Donation is highly supported by the denomination.

BAPTIST

Though Baptists generally believe that organ and tissue donation and transplantation are ultimately matters of personal conscience, the nation's largest Protestant denomination, at their Southern Baptist Convention, adopted a resolution in 1988 encouraging physicians to request organ donation in appropriate circumstances and to "…encourage volunteerism regarding organ donations in the spirit of stewardship, compassion for the needs of others and alleviating suffering." Other Baptist groups have supported organ and tissue donation as an act of charity and leave the decision to donate up to the individual.

BRETHREN

While no official position has been taken by the Brethren denominations, according to Pastor Mike Smith, there is a consensus among the National Fellowship of Grace Brethren that organ and tissue donation is a charitable act so long as it does not impede the life or hasten the death of the donor or does not come from an unborn child.

BUDDHISM

Buddhists believe that organ and tissue donation is a matter of individual conscience and place high value on acts of compassion. Reverend Gyomay Masao, president and founder of the Buddhist Temple of Chicago, says, "We honor those people who donate their bodies and organs to the advancement of medical science and to saving lives." The importance of letting loved ones know one's wishes is stressed.

CATHOLICISM

Catholics view organ and tissue donation as an act of charity and love. Transplants are morally and ethnically acceptable to the Vatican. According to Father Leroy Wickowski, Director of the Office of Health Affairs of the Archdiocese of Chicago, "We encourage donation as an act of charity. It is something good that can result from tragedy and a way for families to find comfort by helping others." Pope John Paul II stated, "The Catholic Church would promote the fact that there is a need for organ donors and that Christians should accept this as a 'challenge to their generosity and fraternal love' so long as ethical principles are followed."

Pope Benedict XVI states: "To donate one's organs is an act of love that is morally licit as long as it is free and spontaneous. To be an organ donor means to carry out an act of love toward someone in need, toward a brother in difficulty. It is a free act of love, of availability, that every person of good will can do at any time and for any brother. As for myself, I have agreed to give my organs to whoever might be in need."

CHRISTIAN CHURCH (DISCIPLES OF CHRIST)

The Christian Church encourages organ and tissue donation, stating that we were created for God's glory and for sharing God's love. A 1985 resolution, adopted by the General Assembly, encourages "members of the Christian Church (Disciples of Christ) to enroll as organ donors and prayerfully support those who have received an organ transplant."

CHRISTIAN SCIENCE

The Church of Christ Scientist does not have a specific position regarding organ donation. According to the First Church of Christ Scientist in Boston, Christian Scientists normally rely on spiritual instead of medical means of healing. They are free, however, to choose whatever form of medical treatment they desire—including a transplant. The question of organ and tissue donation is an individual decision.

CHURCH OF CHRIST (INDEPENDENT)

Generally they have no opposition to organ and tissue donation. Each church is autonomous and leaves the decision to donate up to the individual.

EPISCOPAL

The Episcopal Church passed a resolution in 1982 that recognizes the life-giving benefits of organ, blood and tissue donation. All Christians are encouraged to become organ, blood and tissue donors "…as part of their ministry to others in the name of Christ, who gave His life that we may have life in its fullness."

GYPSIES

Gypsies are a people of different ethnic groups without a formalized religion. They share common folk beliefs and tend to be opposed to organ donation. Their opposition is connected with their beliefs about the afterlife. Traditional belief contends that for a year after death the soul retraces its steps. Thus, the body must remain intact because the soul maintains its physical shape.

HINDUISM

According to the Hindu Temple Society of North America, Hindus are not prohibited by religious law from donating their organs. This act is an individual's decision. H.L. Trivedi, in *Transplantation Proceedings*, states, "Hindu mythology has stories in which the parts of the human body are used for the benefit of other humans and society. There is nothing in the Hindu religion indicating that parts of humans, dead or alive, cannot be used to alleviate the suffering of other humans."

INDEPENDENT CONSERVATIVE EVANGELICAL

Generally, Evangelicals have no opposition to organ and tissue donation. Each church is autonomous and leaves the decision to donate up to the individual.

ISLAM

The religion of Islam believes in the principle of saving human lives. According to A. Sachedina in his *Transplantation Proceedings* (1990) article, "Islamic View on Organ Transplantation," "...the majority of the Muslim scholars belonging to various schools of Islamic Law have invoked the principle of priority of saving human life and have permitted the organ transplant as a necessity to procure that noble end."

JEHOVAH'S WITNESSES

According to the Watch Tower Society, Jehovah's Witnesses believe donation is a matter of individual decision. Jehovah's Witnesses are often assumed to be opposed to donation because of their belief against blood transfusion. However, this merely means that all blood must be removed from the organs and tissues before they are transplanted.

JUDAISM

All four branches of Judaism (Orthodox, Conservative, Reform and Reconstructionist) support and encourage donation. According to Orthodox Rabbi Moses Tendler, chairman of the biology department of Yeshiva University in New York City and chairman of the Bioethics Commission of the Rabbinical Council of America, "If one is in the position to donate an organ to save another's life, it's obligatory to do so, even if the donor never knows who the beneficiary will be. The basic principle of Jewish ethics—'the infinite worth of the human being'— also includes donation of corneas, since eyesight restoration is considered a life-saving operation." In 1991, The Rabbinical Council of America (Orthodox) approved organ donations as permissible, and even required, from brain-dead patients. The Reform movement looks upon the transplant program favorably, and Rabbi Richard Address, director of the Union of American Hebrew Congregation Bio-Ethics Committee and Committee on Older Adults, states that "Judaic Response materials provide a position approach and by and large the North American Reform Jewish community approves of transplantation."

LUTHERAN

In 1984, the Lutheran Church in America passed a resolution stating that donation contributes to the well-being of humanity and can be "an expression of sacrificial love for a neighbor in need." They call on members to consider donating organs and to make any necessary family and legal arrangements, including the use of a signed donor card.

MENNONITE

Mennonites have no formal position on donation, but are not opposed to it. They believe the decision to donate is up to the individual and/or his or her family.

MORAVIAN

The Moravian Church has made no statement addressing organ and tissue donation or transplantation. Robert E. Sawyer, President, Provincial Elders Conference, Moravian Church of America, Southern Province, states, "There is nothing in our doctrine or policy that would prevent a Moravian pastor from assisting a family in making a decision to donate or not to donate an organ." It is, therefore, a matter of individual choice.

MORMON (CHURCH OF JESUS CHRIST OF LATTER DAY SAINTS)

The Church of Jesus Christ of Latter-Day Saints believes that the decision to donate is an individual one made in conjunction with family, medical personnel and prayer. They do not oppose donation.

PENTECOSTAL

Pentecostals believe that the decision to donate should be left up to the individual.

PRESBYTERIAN

Presbyterians encourage and support donation. They respect a person's right to make decisions regarding his or her own body.

SEVENTH-DAY ADVENTIST

Donation and transplantation are strongly encouraged by Seventh-Day Adventists. They have many transplant hospitals, including Loma

Linda in California. Loma Linda specializes in pediatric heart transplantation.

SHINTO

In Shinto, the dead body is considered to be impure and dangerous, and thus quite powerful. "In folk belief context, injuring a dead body is a serious crime…" according to E. Namihira in his article, "Shinto Concept Concerning the Dead Human Body." "Today it is difficult to obtain consent from bereaved families for organ donation or dissection for medical education or pathological anatomy… the Japanese regard them all in the sense of injuring a dead body." Families are often concerned that they not injure the *itai*, the relationship between the dead person and the bereaved people.

SOCIETY OF FRIENDS (QUAKERS)

Organ and tissue donation is believed to be an individual decision. The Society of Friends does not have an official position on donation.

UNITARIAN UNIVERSALIST

Organ and tissue donation is widely supported by Unitarian Universalists. They view it as an act of love and selfless giving.

UNITED CHURCH OF CHRIST

Reverend Jay Lintner, Director, Washington Office of the United Church of Christ Office for Church in Society, states, "United Church of Christ people, churches and agencies are extremely and overwhelmingly supportive of organ sharing. The General Synod has never spoken to this issue because, in general, the Synod speaks on more controversial issues, and there is no controversy about organ sharing, just as there is no controversy about blood donation. Blood donation rooms have been set up at several General Synods. Similarly, any organized effort to get the General Synod delegates or individual churches to sign organ donation cards would meet with generally positive responses."

UNITED METHODIST

The United Methodist Church issued a policy statement regarding organ and tissue donation. In it they state that "The United Methodist Church recognizes the life-giving benefits of organ and tissue donation, and thereby encourages all Christians to become organ and tissue donors by signing and carrying cards or driver's licenses, attesting their commitment of such organs upon their death, to those in need, as part of their ministry to others in the name of Christ, who gave his life that we might have life in its fullness." *Book of Resolutions 2000*, page 352. See also 162U Social Principles: Organ Transplantation and Donation, *Book of Discipline 2000*, page 112.